THE GAY KAMA SUTRA

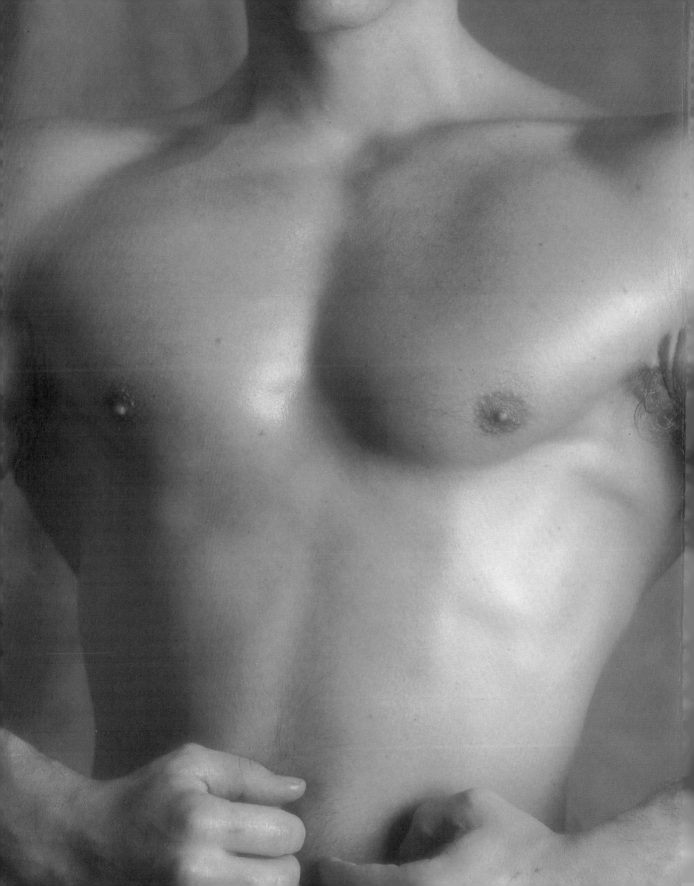

THE GAY KAMA SUTRA

COLIN SPENCER

St. Martin's Press   New York.

First published in the United Kingdom 1996
Copyright © Labyrinth Publishing (UK) Ltd 1996
Texrt Copyright © Colin Spencer 1996

The right of Colin Spencer to be identified as the author of the work has been
asserted by him in accordance with the Copyright, Design and Patents Act, 1988.

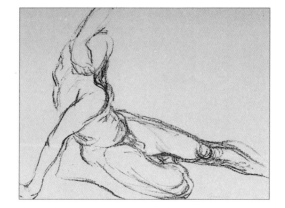

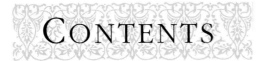

CONTENTS

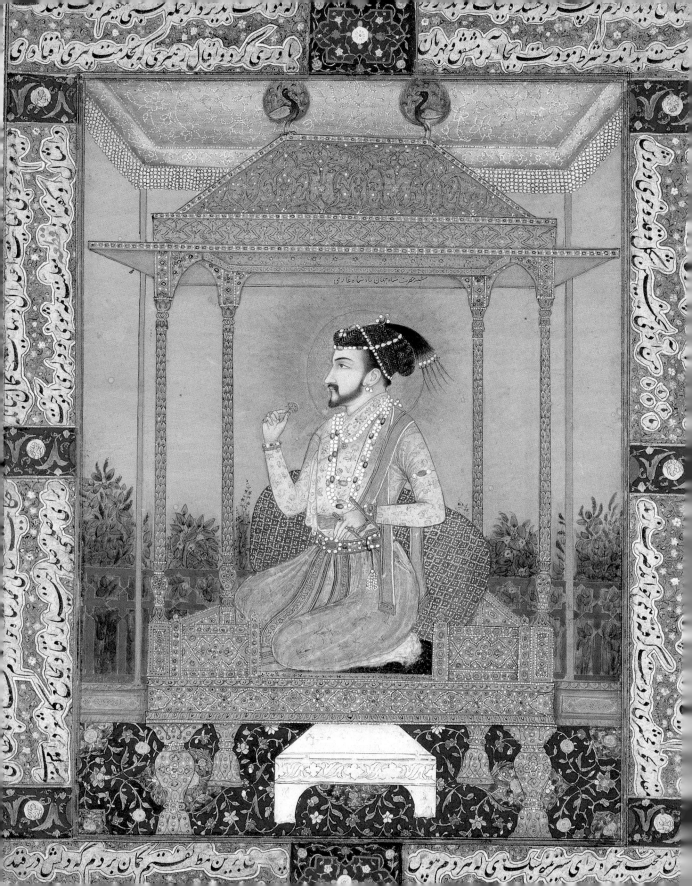

INTRODUCTION

The *Kama Sutra* is a manual for love and life, written in India in the fourth century A.D. It exhorts the reader, enthusiastically and passionately, to celebrate sexual pleasure as one of the highest of all human experiences. It is lavish in its commands to enjoy the flesh; it is elaborate in its instructions on how to practice sex in myriad ways; it is positive and joyful in its approach. Designed with the intention of teaching young people about human sexuality, *The Kama Sutra* offers a clear and simple understanding of this most intimate side of our nature.

Various parts of *The Kama Sutra* were gathered between the third and first centuries B.C., then six authors worked upon it further: Charayana, Suvarnanagha, Ghotakamukha, Gonardiya, Godnikaputra and Dattaka. Their compilations, which described the customs of the Maurya period of the fourth century B.C., were updated eight hundred years later in the fourth century A.D. by a Brahman "man of letters," Vatsyayana. It was this work that became popular and that was eventually translated into English by Richard Burton and F.F. Arbuthnot, who created the Kama Shastra Society for the express purpose of publishing works of eroticism, such as Burton's translation of *The Arabian Nights. The Kama Sutra* was first published in English in 1883. No translators' names were given when it appeared, so delicate and controversial was it deemed to be. Instead the book bore the name of the Kama Shastra Society of London and Benares. (*Kama* is Sanskrit for "love, pleasure, sensual gratification;" *Shastra* means "scripture" or "doctrines;" *Sutra* means "aphorisms" or "compressed expressions using the minimum of words.") An apt translation of *The Kama Sutra* could be "The Rules of Love." The whole work is composed of very

Opposite: Shah Jahan, the seventeenth-century Mughal emperor who built love's greatest shrine, the Taj Mahal.

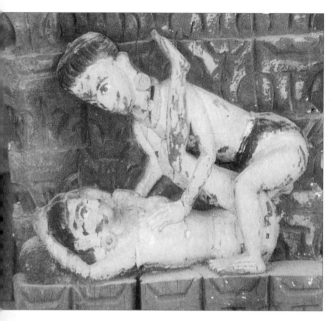

Male coupling. A sixteenth-century wood carving from the Hanuman Temple in Kathmandu, Nepal. The monkey god Hanuman, celebrated for his sexual prowess, was the focus of exclusively male cults.

Running heads: Banquet scene from a fifth-century B.C. Greek tomb at Paestum, southern Italy, showing youths playing *kottabos*, in which wine is thrown into a bowl.

succinct directions on the manner in which life may be enjoyed to the full.

Vatsyayana wrote at the end of the work that he had composed the treatise "according to the precepts of the Holy Writ" and that the work "was not to be used merely as an instrument for satisfying our desires." Indeed, it was treated as a great sacred work on spiritual life, how men and women should behave to become good citizens and devoted followers of the gods. Not for one moment was *The Kama Sutra* thought to be pornographic; only in the nineteenth century was it considered so. And the notion that sex is surrounded by guilt or inhibition is nowhere expressed. The work is a hymn to life's pleasures, for in ancient Hinduism there was a unity between the life of the spirit and that of the flesh. To make love with finesse and tenderness was to imitate the creators, to mirror the gods in the most divine act. Sexuality engendered both awe and respect, and sex was seen as the human counterpoint to divine creation, as a sacrament. But sexuality was also openly expressed, normal, necessary, and the most intense pleasure in life.

The original *Kama Sutra* was, therefore, not just a book of sexual techniques; it was also a guide to how a man may conduct himself in society; how, observing the customs of the time, he may relate to his peers. It indicates both the vast differences in social customs between India of the fourth century and our own age, and at the same time the symmetry of the two societies' respective experiences and knowledge of sexual pleasure. As *The Kama Sutra* is timeless in its advice on sexuality, and encompasses all aspects of love, it can be used equally well by gay men today: everything it says of male and female love-making can be applied to two gay men; and it can provide advice on lifestyle and the problems of being gay in a society which is equivocal and often downright prejudiced about homosexuality. *The Kama Sutra's* joyful and uninhibited approach to sensuality in all its richness, its connection of fleshly pleasure to all else in life, should be adopted and

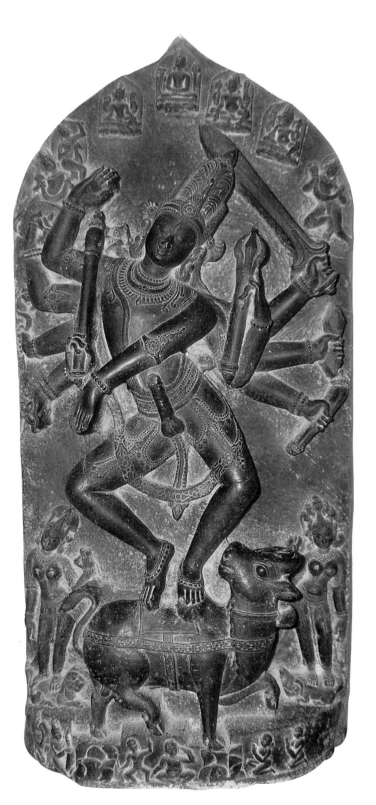

Shiva, the Creator God of the
Hindu pantheon, dancing atop
the bull Nandi, symbolizing
the conquest of the ego.

encouraged time and time again, especially by a sexual minority which is oppressed in so many parts of the world and which has only lately—and very grudgingly in Judeo-Christian cultures—found a modicum of acceptance.

Taken as a whole, the original *Kama Sutra* would be a bizarre model for today's world. At least two-thirds of it has little direct relevance to modern society, either straight or gay, because it concerns the manners and customs of a time and culture whose view of human beings is vastly different from our own. It is highly elitist, as indeed was the society that conceived it, and permeated by the ethos of the caste system. Restrictions are placed upon what a person may do, and with whom. The men do no work of any kind: they are rich, and spend their days in an endless round of diversions dedicated to pleasure and to pleasurable learning, which embraces the arts, sciences, and theology. The book clearly states that the more learned and skilled a man is in these fine arts, the better he is considered as a lover.

Ancient works of literature show a high regard for civilized values, but are dismissive of the working people (the majority, after all) who upheld the very civilization the elite were smugly praising. The workers were not regarded or acknowledged, any more than, for example, Victorian servants who waited at table within earshot of all sorts of personal intimacies. The members of this underclass had no rights; they were thought to be barely human, and no ideology ever illumined their plight.

The Kama Sutra is very precise about who is not to be sexually enjoyed: women who are extremely white or extremely black, as well as lepers, lunatics, ascetics, and female friends. So among these, racial and sexual prejudice (upon which the caste system was partly based, and still is) is a further example of its lack of humanity. Nowadays we ourselves decide what constitutes an acceptable partner, and many of our sexual contacts are friends.

Notwithstanding, it would be inappropriate to dismiss *The Kama Sutra* because it lacks humanity or political correctness by modern perceptions. The work must be accepted on its own terms, and with it the many "blind spots" of the ancient seers.

The main and most significant theme of *The Kama Sutra* is its positive and enthusiastic approach to erotic delights. Much of the original

Opposite: Shah Jahan, portrayed as the essence of cultivated Indian nobility.

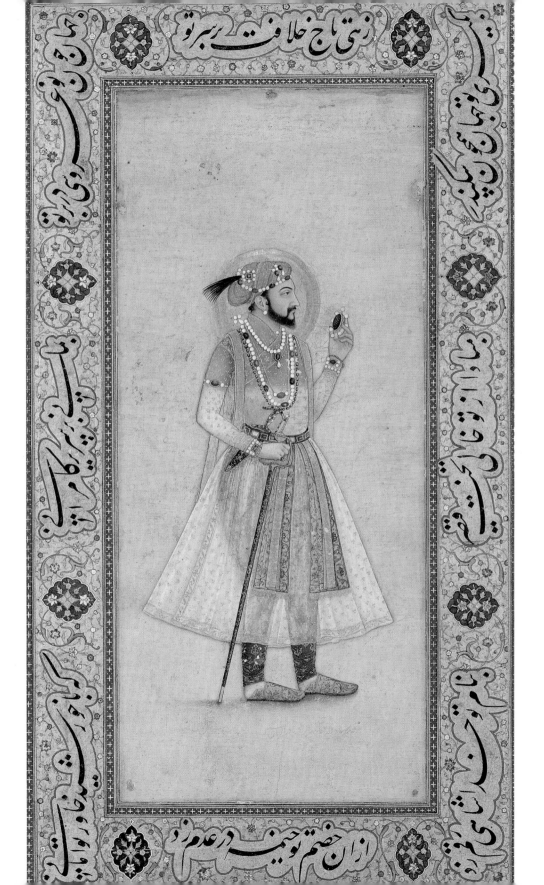

11

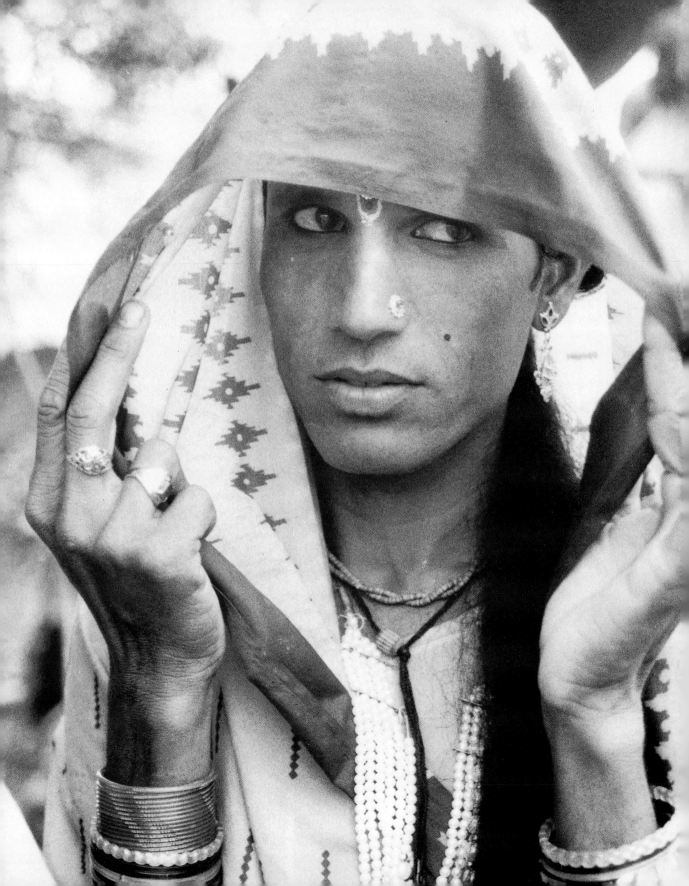

work is concerned with instilling the right attitudes to love-making in the male: how he should approach the female, how he should relax her, and the various types of foreplay that he can use to encourage her to respond. Then there are the descriptions of all the positions that can be employed in the sexual act. *The Kama Sutra* shows us that nothing (or very little) new can be revealed about sex; it also indicates that in the last two thousand years we have allowed Christian notions to destroy much of our spontaneous pleasure in the natural desires of our own bodies.

In *The Kama Sutra* all sexual positions are described and all orifices are used in intercourse. Tantric texts emphasized the significance of the anus, which was considered one of the most important centers of psychic energy, and supported a strong belief in the mystical power of semen. These positive aspects make the work very relevant to the gay world today. All gay people living under the shadow of AIDS should be familiar with it.

Much of *The Kama Sutra*, however, denigrates gay society. For example, gay sex is not even mentioned in a mixed *ménage á trois*. It is treated briefly and unsympathetically in the context of eunuchs, who are referred to as the "third sex." Here is an excerpt from the *Auparishtaka* (Superior Coition, or Fellatio):

Those of the third sex with a feminine appearance imitate women in their whole manner of being. They dress themselves and their hair in female fashion, imitating women's speech and laughter, their dragging gait, flirting and silliness, their sweetness, gentleness, hesitation, patience and modesty, and take up women's amusements.

They perform the act that takes place between the thighs in the mouth, which is why it is called superior coition.

Those that like men but dissimulate the fact maintain a manly appearance and earn their living as hairdressers or masseurs. They practise oral coition, but their sexual desires are dissimulated, since they appear masculine.

During the practice of massage, the masseur rests his body against that of the man and kneads his thighs on the side of his intimate parts (upuguha). He draws his face closer to the man's thighs as he kneads them.

Opposite: A devotee of the god Krishna at the religious festival of Kumbh Mela at Nashik, north of Bombay. The Hindu transvestite tradition continues in northern India today.

13

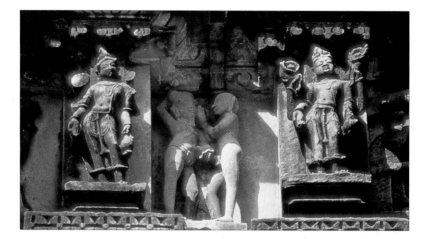

Eleventh-century red stone temple carvings from Khajuraho in Madhya Pradesh, India, showing a sexual encounter between an older and a younger man. They are flanked by a pair of male gods. Many strands of the Hindu Shaiv tradition were for male initiates only.

Continuing his investigation, he touches the sexual area at the thigh joint, he draws his face closer to the man's thighs as he kneads them. He then touches the sexual area; ignoring the penis, he touches the balls (jaghanabhaga) then when he manages to provoke an erection, he takes the penis in his hand, strokes it and, audaciously he commences action, sucking without being asked to.

This passage presents gay people as silly and hesitant, with a dragging gait, among other things, suggesting that they were as despised and marginalized as they are in our own society. This excerpt is no more than a description of a blow job in a massage parlor. No poetry is read, no love songs are sung, no lute is played or chessmen set out. In short, the paraphernalia of love, which is described in such detail in the rest of the work when men and women are involved, is wholly absent.

That gay sex gets such short shrift is strange, considering the great pantheon of Hindu gods and goddesses, which include hermaphroditic, transvestite and other deities that change their sex at will. Their Supreme Being, after all, was thought to possess both male and female principles, while Tantrism taught that every man has in him a female element and every woman a masculine element. Sex for Hindus did not exist just for procreation (for which the Christian religion restricted it), and could be engaged in for pleasure, for power, and even for magic. Sex was also allied with mysticism: copulation was one method of getting in touch with deeper layers of consciousness, and thereby understanding the mysteries of existence. One of the great secrets gay people must embrace is that *The Kama Sutra* points out and emphasizes this link.

The penis itself was often worshiped, the phallus of the guru kissed and adored. Phalluses were worn about the neck, while all kinds of dildoes made from candle-wax, baked clay, bone or wood were used by both men and women to give themselves pleasure. Masturbation was enthusiastically recommended in *The Kama Sutra*, for Krishna himself was believed to practise manual orgasm. Mothers stimulated the penises of their infants and gave a "deep massage" to their daughters as a form of affectionate consolation. (In China in the Ming period, when kissing on the lips was thought obscene, mothers would kiss the penises of their infant sons.) A fixed stone phallus in a secluded part of the temple served for the ritual deflowering of girls.

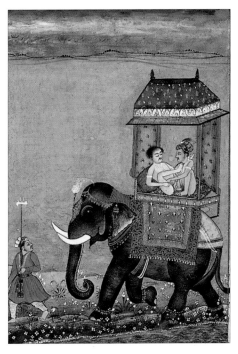

A contemporary Indian homoerotic miniature in the Mughal tradition.

India has a long tradition of male prostitution. As late as 1948, when India achieved independence, some Hindu temples still had women and boy prostitutes. In the cities of northern India groups of male transvestite or transsexual devotees of the Mother Goddess (Parvati, Bachuchara Mata) sing, dance and beg for alms. They, too, also engage in homosexual prostitution.

Today India is not as tolerant as it once was. Though homosexual transvestites are accepted as dancers and entertainers in all the major cities, social support of gay and lesbian rights is nearly non-existent. Homosexual acts between men are illegal, with a maximum penalty of life imprisonment or a fine. There have been reports of raids in Bombay and arrests being made of men because they look homosexual. They are fined or beaten with laths on the road outside the police station. This is deeply depressing, given India's past and the great sexual worth of the *Kama Sutra.*

Perhaps today's intolerance stems from the same reason that gay love is largely ignored in the *Kama Sutra*: though the ancient society was entirely male-dominated,

15

it was based upon the concept of unity between the *lingam* (phallus) and the *yoni* (vagina). For example, the union of *Purusha* (matter) and *Prakroto* (energy) was symbolized by the union of Shiva (*lingam*) and Shakti (*yoni*). Though the feminine side of the male was clearly embodied by Shiva, who was half-woman, no union between *lingam* and *lingam* was envisaged, this being merely a conflict of matter with matter. However, as the anal orifice was regarded with such respect as a center of psychic energy, it is surprising that a unity of matter and energy was not joyfully celebrated there.

The most striking contrast between *The Kama Sutra's* fourth-century Indian perspective and that of Western society today is apparent in the differing concepts of masculinity. In our society, great emphasis is placed on "manliness," which is defined as heterosexual aggression, as dominance, power, and triumph. An anthropologist examining this concept might come to the conclusion that the straight male in Western culture is a puny, insecure individual who needs to boost his failing virility with myths of sexual power rather as the Samurai did when, during their declining influence in Japanese society, they had themselves portrayed with massive cocks.

Ancient India's ideal male is a highly educated poet, whose clothes and rooms are beautifully decorated and perfumed, who teaches parrots to talk, who sings and plays on the lute, who studies the characters in Hindu drama, and who diverts himself and his companions by pelting them with flowers. The high point of his year is the festival of the goddess Saraswati, the patroness of the fine arts, and especially of music and rhetoric, which included harmony, eloquence and language. In fact, much of *The Kama Sutra's* ancient advice to heterosexual men might today find a more sympathetic and interested hearing from gay men.

The order and subjects of the chapters in this book follow those of the original *Kama Sutra*. Chapter One reflects fourth-century India's emphasis upon the metaphysics of love and its exhortation to be skilled in the arts and sciences. Chapter Two deals with the art of sexual love-making; many positions are described here, reflecting much of the original, but adapted to gay lovers today. Chapter Three deals with male sexuality and the society we live in (any book on gay sex has to address both of these components). Chapter Four explores sexual

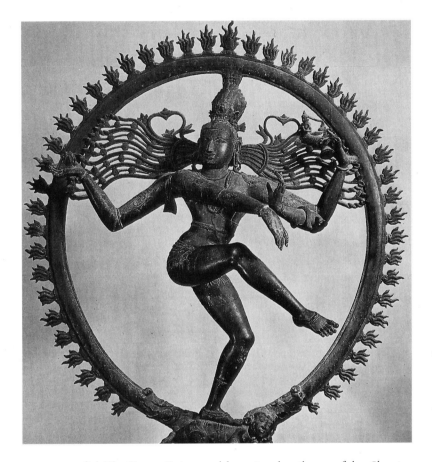

Shiva Nataraja, Lord of the Dance, through which he performs the creation of the universe. A twelfth-century bronze statue from south India.

games, as did *The Kama Sutra*, and how to play them safely. Chapter Five advises the reader on acquiring a partner. Chapter Six gives a list of aphrodisiacs and essential oils suitable for romantic uses.

The Gay Kama Sutra has been written with great respect for the original. It is also a passionate plea to promote gay love in all its depth and ecstasy and, especially, the ongoing struggle for justice and equality in today's society.

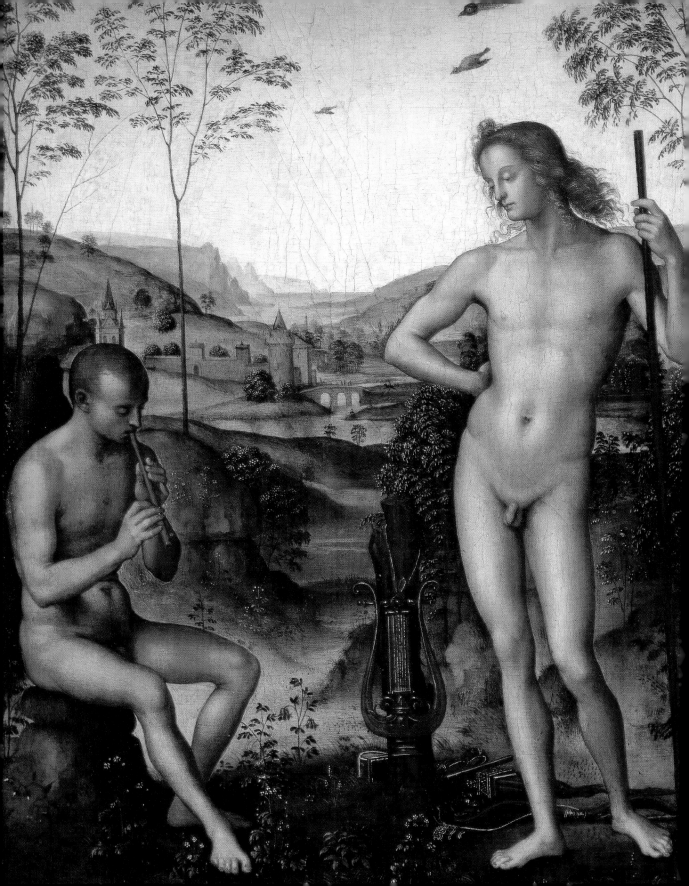

CHAPTER ONE

THE ART OF LOVE

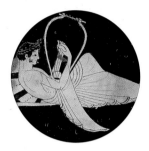

The art of love is the center of life, because it draws its great power from all else in life. Our extrovert world, composed of all the familiar forms, the Earth and its skies and all the breathing creatures within it, exudes a secret language which we have now forgotten, but which we begin to recollect in the act of love.

Love cannot be fulfilled within a vacuum. Love is illuminated by the world's entity, that concept of complete wholeness which is constantly recreating itself, which springs into sentient life within the known world.

Every man is on Earth to symbolize something he is ignorant of and to realize a particle or a mountain of the invisible materials that will serve to build the City of Nirvana.

All of this creation reflects, as in a mirror, that which is unknown, veiled from us and thereby mysterious. Thus, the act of love combines both worlds, unites the known and the unknown, which is the reason for its great magical powers.

No one knows what he has come into this world to do, what his acts correspond to, his sentiments, his ideas, or what his real name is, his enduring Name in the Register of Light. Yet, in the act of true love, he begins to discern the mysterious truths of what is never finally revealed to him.

Thus, in order to perfect the art of love, our knowledge of the hidden world must become more acute, while the act of love itself must be placed within the context of life as it is lived.

This manual attempts to embrace the spiritual exercises and the living

Opposite: Apollo, Greek god of the Sun and of Music, and Marsyas, the Phrygian flute-player, painted by Perugino (1446-1523). Classical mythology was always a good excuse for portraying the Renaissance delight in the male nude.

Above: Painting of a youth playing a lyre on a Greek bowl of the sixth century B.C.

skills by which we can relate to each other, addressing itself to the problems which are hindrances to our happiness and to the happiness of others.

THE AIMS OF LIFE

The principal aim of life is to be perfect in love, but to achieve this perfection a man has first of all to be true to his inner self. We must, therefore, listen closely to the inner voices and follow their lead, for they will show us the path toward fulfillment. We may be embarking upon a long journey with no foreseeable end, the road may curve and wind, the path may seem blocked and hazardous, but the significant step is the step that moves onward. The purpose is to keep on traveling, even through darkness, while always attempting to listen to the silence, to hear those secret voices within us.

When the individual reaches fulfillment, he does not realize his state of perfection. For the Self can never be aware of its fulfillment. But others will be aware of the journey that he has undergone and they will admire and love the serenity within him. They will admire and love the strength of purpose that he brings to all things and the dexterity of skills and calm persuasion that are implicit in the gift that we call love. For the fulfilled man will be one of those who love the world in all its complexity and rich array, both the exterior and the interior worlds, which lesser souls mistakenly believe are always in conflict. Thus, this manual is to teach men to become perfect in love, skilled in all things, to be unafraid of all things, to be sensitive to the gift of life, to learn its secrets and to live them tenderly as an opening flower bud.

After a man has attained being true to himself, his second aim is to listen with great attention to others, to learn to be sensitive to their inner voices, to learn to hear their voices even when they themselves are attempting to drown them out with their own sound and fury. Great love can erase all ephemeral sound, allowing the enlightened man to concentrate upon the truth.

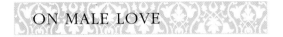

ON MALE LOVE

Throughout history the penis has been revered as an organ of great beauty and power. In the ancient world there were many stone phalluses which were objects of worship. There were many rituals in ancient religions in which men venerated the phallus and made love to each other, or virgin youths were deflowered, or male priests fellated the King. Many myths tell of great gods that drank semen to become indestructible.

Male love is as old as civilization itself. It flowered because it was a rite of passage for boys in becoming youths and youths in becoming men. It was a total love which included sexual love as part of a respected social structure. Male love was used to teach values to a young man ready to take his position in a community.

Male love flourished when women were set apart as mothers to nurture the hierarchical line. Sexual pleasure was taken outside the marital bed, and because girls had to keep their virginity until marriage for motherhood, boys and youths were favored.

Male love has always been with us, at the center of all communities, whether it is celebrated or suppressed, whether it is an honored part of the culture of a society or pushed into an underworld. All men need to realize the ancient tradition of gay loving and never be ashamed of their own sexual nature. Unless men are released from shame and guilt, they cannot give love freely. Shame and guilt are hidden poisons that will slowly destroy the integrity and pride in a man. Free yourself of all notions of inferiority. This is an essential part of becoming a whole man.

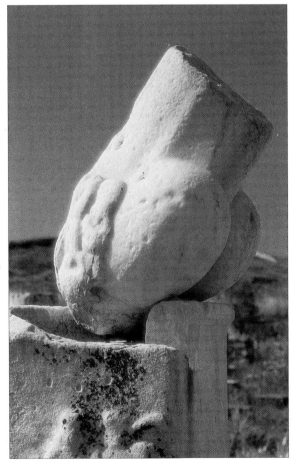

The remains of a phallus along the sacred way of the temples on the island of Delos, Greece. The ancient world felt awe and reverence for the phallus and enjoyed representing it.

THE THREE COMPONENTS OF LIFE

Perfect love-making starts in the mind. The curious mind is always enquiring into the reason. In love we learn about others, and in others we learn the secrets that we often do not care to know about ourselves. In the life of our lover we can imagine what we are to become, and we always have the choice of whether to dwell there or not.

The most fulfilling love-making springs from a harmony of flesh, spirit and mind. These elements relate to the three worlds within us: *kama*, *dharma* and *artha*. Each one of us can attempt to achieve this harmony by exercising these three worlds throughout our lives.

The three worlds may be defined thus:

Kama—a combination of sensuality and sensitivity, a heightening of all the five senses, so that hearing, seeing, taste, smelling and feeling are all energized and invigorated. All these senses should combine in the act of love.

Dharma—an appreciation of the ultimate mystery in all things. A humility and an awe felt in response to the vastness of time and creation. A religious sense which should be intensified in the act of love, for in this act you are as one with the divine creator.

Artha—a sense of social responsibility, being just to others and fair to yourself. If this exterior world is not correct then neither the soul nor the flesh can be at peace with itself. An explicit component of a man's *artha* today is the struggle for equality in the campaign against gay discrimination.

The aims of life might be described as an exploration of all three worlds, a journey taken throughout all three. As infants it is *kama* only that we know at first. All of our senses react with surprise and joy as we learn the characteristics of the world around and within us. Then as small children we become aware of *dharma*, the vast infinity of creation itself, and first learn to wonder at it. At the same time we begin to learn the nature of *artha*, its demands on us, our place in the social order, and to understand our connection with others. As we travel through all three worlds, our task is to balance our awareness of them. When in danger of becoming overpowered by one of them, we must never forget the existence of the others.

Some people might criticize such claims, saying that *dharma* has nothing to do with sexuality, and is indeed at war with it, for the world of the spirit can only be eroded by sexual desire. By sacrificing sexual desire the world of the spirit is enhanced.

Those who believe that love of the flesh is in conflict with the spirit make a tragic assumption which springs from fear of both the flesh and the unknown. Sexual pleasure alone can lead a man into distress, lead him to commit unrighteous deeds, make him indifferent to the future and encourage a laxity in all else. But sexual love combined with an appreciation of all spiritual values enhances both the flesh and the spirit.

Others argue, how can the practice of *artha* influence the happy gratification of sexual love, when all of us have known great lovers who have refused to make any gifts towards it?

Love is best given from a whole man who is at peace with himself. Anger makes a poor lover. Anger, bitterness and envy all spring from a man who has hidden from the demands of *artha*. Perhaps you have called a man a great lover because he is lustful and has many orgasms, but such a man has given himself up to pleasure alone, and in middle age will be ruined and lonely.

Courtier and servants of the
Raja Patalia, Delhi, *c*.1817

THE ACQUISITION OF KNOWLEDGE

The more we know, the greater our respect for all life. Therefore, the arts and sciences should be studied. If we value creation itself, we learn to value the individual. The greater a man's learning, the more entertaining his conversation, the sharper his wit, the more perceptive his judgments. The educated man is able to give others great riches of mind and spirit. Finally, true learning bestows wisdom, the wisdom which shows us the magnitude of our ignorance, the vastness of our lack of knowledge. In the wise man's perception of others there is always understanding, and in his loving there is always kindness.

The following should be studied, though it would be a polymath and a genius who could know them all:

~ Music; both to sing and to play on all kinds of instruments. To listen attentively to all forms of song and musical drama.

~ Movement and dance; both practicing all forms of dance and attending performances of the most superlative kind.

~ Astronomy; to study the stars and planets and the whole mysterious universe and to read the news of its new-found secrets.

~ Knowledge of dictionaries and vocabularies.

The practice of handwriting, so that notes and letters can be sent to the beloved. Nothing is more illuminating than the written script of the beloved; this should not only be always aesthetically pleasing, but should honestly reflect the character and aspirations of the writer. A handsome hand-written script involves flexibility and control over the arm, wrist, hand and fingers. Movement exercises for these parts of the body are beneficial.

The same exercises are essential for skill in drawing, which requires a fusion between eye and hand. To be able to capture reality in this way is a talent that can be sharpened by practice and can give much pleasure to others.

~ Tattooing is another form of drawing; this enhances the body.
~ Coloring the hair, nails and teeth. Coloring parts of the body and adorning those parts with beads, rings, necklaces of glass, pearls and colored stones, feathers, leather and gold buckles.
~ The art of weaving cloth and making lace.
~ The art of making money by being honest and just in the affairs of all men.
~ The art of building dwellings, both simple and complicated.

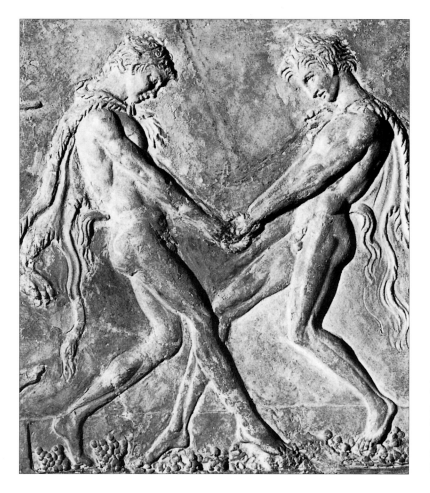

Youths dancing during the grape harvest. A terracotta relief from the fourth century B.C. The Greeks imbued all daily acts with undisguised sensuality.

~ The art of designing fountains, waterfalls, streams, lakes and ponds, then filling them with flowers, plants and fish.

~ Designing the apartment or living quarters, arranging beds and couches with coverings of soft rugs and cushions, lighting these areas subtly.

~ Decorating these same areas with paintings, flowers, silks, glassware and china, so that a harmonious whole is achieved.

~ The art of cooking beautiful, appetizing and tempting dishes which contain no parts of any dead animals. The eating of dead flesh lumbers the spirit with the ghosts of past tragedies and long misery.

~ The art of spices, their tastes and aromas, so as not only to flavor these dishes but perfume the flesh and the air with subtle but

25

intense aromatics that seduce the spirit and flesh of the beloved.

~ The art of aromatherapy, to be able to use many perfumes and unguents so as to be able to massage the flesh of the beloved with a tender and delicate touch.

Exercise at the gymnasium, so as to allow the body to perform many difficult physical maneuvers with grace and beauty, but not to let the concept of the body beautiful override all else: though the body should be lithe and well proportioned, both the mind and the spirit must be equally well trained. Balance in all things is the key, and must never be forgotten.

The art of gardening, in which the very first essential is to understand the soil and to enrich it over the years with rich humus as occurs naturally in the depth of the forest. Then to respect the plant and to till the soil delicately upon the surface so that all its secrets may be kept hidden, and to use only natural products in such gardening, as was done from the earliest of days.

Languages and the roots of language and to be able to speak fluently in many countries, but always to respect cultures which may be alien, to know their manners and customs and to observe them with particularity. Behavior toward other cultures must be ruled only by charity and the love of the human condition.

Sensitivity to and the ability to read from the body language of human beings, their gestures and expressions. To be able to read words in a silence, to perceive sense in a wordless sound.

The understanding of the technology of communication, to be fleet with its skills.

The understanding of the technology of movement upon land, air and sea, and to understand and tame the nature of the machine.

Skill in all types of sports and games.

Knowledge of the art of diplomacy.

Knowledge of the customs of society.

Skill in speaking verse.

The names and character of the natural world. To be able to walk in the countryside and reveal all details when such enquiries

Painting of a discus thrower on a Greek bowl. The classical ideal was a sound mind in a sound body.

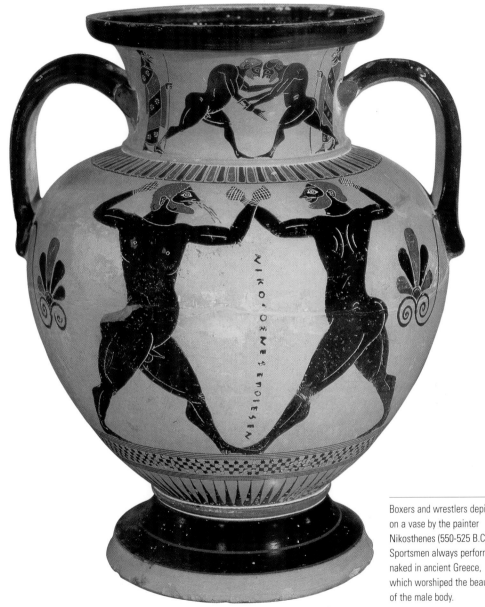

Boxers and wrestlers depicted
on a vase by the painter
Nikosthenes (550-525 B.C).
Sportsmen always performed
naked in ancient Greece,
which worshiped the beauty
of the male body.

might be made of the name of a tree or a plant or a bird.

Respect for all living creatures with which we share the planet. To understand that we are caught in the same net of time and space as they are, and that they have gifts of intuition, knowledge and perception that we can never learn or share.

The art of nursing, to nurture the ill, sick, and dying. To tend animals with the same tenderness as humans.

A man who is adept at a mere ten of these and is endowed with a good disposition, beauty and other winning qualities will achieve a seat of honor in the assembly of men. He will, moreover, be respected by the king and praised by learned men and his favor will be sought by all. He will become an object of universal regard. Nor could he ever lack for suitors keen to beg for his hand. Such a man would have the pick of the choicest and most beautiful young men in the land as his adored concubine. Such a man might sleep with a new lover every night of the year if he did not find such behavior hollow and without true savor. Such a man would wait patiently for his true love.

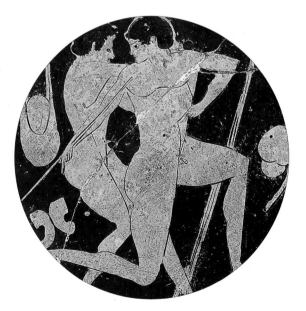

Athletes training. Scene from a Greek bowl, fifth century B.C.

THE CONDUCT OF THE WELL BRED

Cleanliness is essential, so shower and wash the hair every morning first thing, after emptying all waste matter from the body. (Exercise may be taken before such ablutions, the best being to swim naked in the sea.) While showering, wash with perfumed soaps and sing. Shaving the face, if it is necessary or desirable, may be performed next, then rinsing with ice cold water and using modestly aromatic lotions upon the skin in order to increase the smoothness of the lips, chin and cheeks.

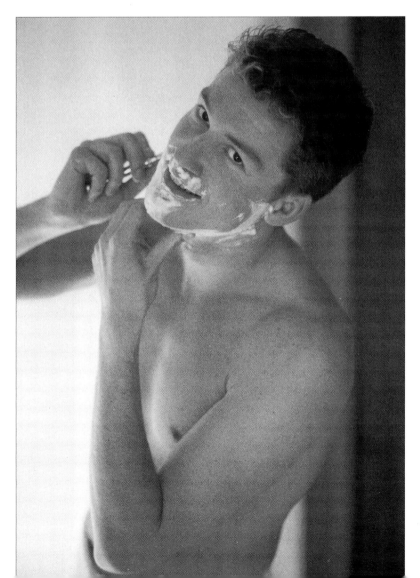

Daily care of the body is part of self-esteem.

29

Next the apparel must always be clean, freshly washed and smelling of air and sunlight. The repast should be light and well-balanced, as in freshly squeezed fruit juices and herbal teas, raw fruits, nuts, vegetables and cereals. Gentle exercise is always important, whether taken while at work or on the way to work.

Be deferential to all colleagues, whatever their status, but also be firm with any who may not return your tact. Have a balanced sense of your own importance, because without that self approximation, which is only another form of self-love, no respect or love can be given to others. Therefore, know yourself well in whatever situation you are in, but continually test what you believe are your limits. The human soul is limitless and we are capable of more things than we can ever imagine. Do not be restricted by others, but be firm in your adventures. Explore all things which at first seem to threaten you or others with you, for the fear that resides in you is the only fear to be overcome. The only evil in this world is that which men believe in and act upon.

If there is a mid-day meal, eat lightly. Fresh fruit juices and raw salads are essential to the body and spirit and give the best nutrition because in them the life-giving minerals and vitamins are at their most intense.

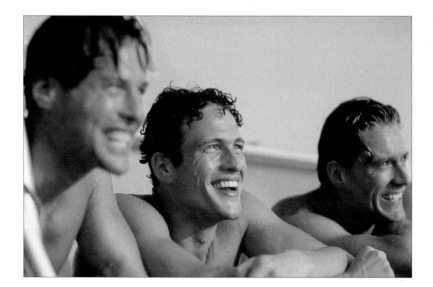

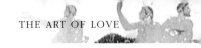

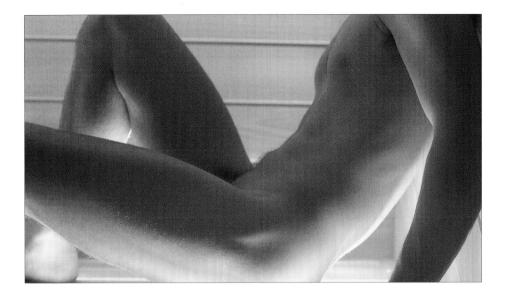

Cleanliness is again vital before the evening. Particular attention may be paid to those areas of the body which contain the most sexual power. Oils and lotions can be massaged gently into the flesh or used for dyeing the pubic hair. Ornaments which give pleasure may be arranged upon the body. Think of the body as an instrument which will be played tenderly to give sweet music.

In relationships, men should tell the truth. Fantasy has its part in play, but everyone should be able to recognize it as such. The truth is the solid ground from which we dream, and without such ground we are rootless: we drift and wander. Without the truth, without being surrounded by people who are dedicated to telling the truth, we are lost. Be firm and ruthless with people who lie, scheme and are full of devious plots. Cut them out of your life, for they cannot be cured, and until you are ruthless such people will cling on like leeches sucking the life blood from you.

Friends are as important as lovers. Lovers should also be friends. Friendships should always be free from envy and covetousness. We should exult in the successes of our friends. To covet what is theirs is to desire to be untrue to oneself.

Truth to one's own nature is the most important secret of all.

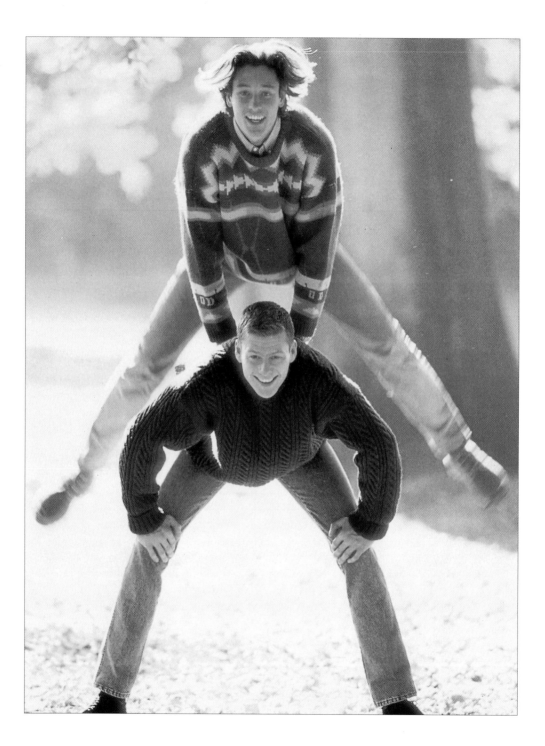

Honesty starts within yourself. Examine yourself and what you have done, what you believe in, what you desire to do. Put aside a small part of the day for such thoughts. If you are unhappy, work out the true cause of your unhappiness, because in knowing the cause we can generally correct the fault.

Beware of both alcohol and drugs, because they distort reality and stretch truth so that it merges into fantasy. To act under their influence is to commit a kind of lie. However, some small amount of both can enlighten the soul, stimulate the spirit and make the tongue lively with wit. If used, they must be in your service. Beware of using either as a crutch for despair, for addiction will quickly make you the servant instead of the master.

Be generous to all people with your warmth and understanding. Listening is a great art. Be polite and discreet, have a sense of what is appropriate at what time, be ingenious and resourceful. Do not push yourself forward in great excitement, rather hang back a little and speak slowly and soberly.

Never allow others to suggest that you are inadequate in any way. If you allow a slight against yourself it is because you must be in agreement with it. Consider this, for people who are mocked are not happy and are used as scapegoats for great and small crimes. Stamp out such behavior in others before it can take hold. Never allow them one gesture or remark that seems superior; crush it instantly as a sign of crude barbarism that stems from little education and understanding.

Left: At the Gay Pride March, London. A new awareness of togetherness has been forged at Gay Pride marches in cities throughout the Western world.

THE LIFE OF A CITIZEN

Having thus acquired learning and an income from work he enjoys, a citizen should become a householder in a city or town and within the vicinity of men with like-minded passions. All the better if the abode is near some water, for the human spirit is elevated by the sight of a sea, river or lake. The abode should be divided into different compartments given over to different purposes. It should be surrounded by garden, and contain at least two rooms, the outer and the inner one. The outer one is for public discourse, for matters of *artha* and for eating and bathing. The inner one should have a soft bed in it, agreeable to the sight, and covered with a clean, white cloth and a canopy garlanded with flowers. The bed will have pillows and cushions piled on it. There should also be a couch, and a stool upon which should be placed the fragrant ointments of the night as well as things used for perfuming the mouth, and flowers and plants in pots, and love verses and books of philosophy to calm the soul. Near the couch on the ground there should be a pot for spitting, a box containing ornaments and jewels, also a lute hanging from an elephant's tooth on which to pluck a melody. Not far from the couch there should be a chessboard and chessmen, a pair of dice, oils for massage, iced water and fruit juices.

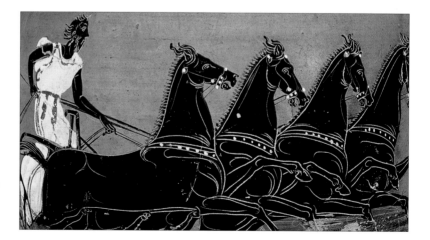

Competitor in a chariot race. Painting on a Greek vase from the fifth century B.C.

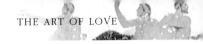

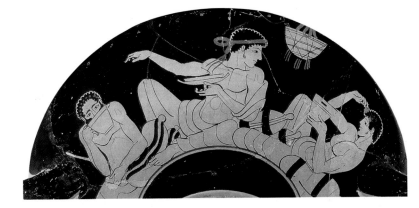

Young men at a banquet,
painted on the underside of a
Greek bowl, *c.*480 B.C.

The following are the five things to be done occasionally as diversions
and amusements.

Festivals

On some particular days throughout the year, citizens assemble to celebrate a festival. There the skills of singers, dancers and actors are
often heard and praised. The good citizen extends warm hospitality to
all strangers on these occasions and conducts himself with due deco-
rum. Diplomacy and politeness must rule the temperament, for the
good citizen should have respect for the feelings of others. Only when
an injustice is seen to be done should he speak out to expose it.

Social gatherings

Men of the same age, disposition and talents, fond of the same diversions and with the same degree of education, may sit together and
engage in agreeable discourse with each other. The subjects of discourse may be a new book or play, a new production of an opera or
many other expressions of the arts or sciences. The talk may eventually turn to love and some new beauty who has turned all heads. In such
a moment it is best to be well served by humor, to stand back from the
human comedy and to observe whether covetousness or true desire is
displayed. Many older men who are accomplished in the ways of the

35

world and respected for their social influence desire only to have a beautiful decoration hanging upon their arm which will reflect well upon them in public. Such men are puffed up with vanity and will surround the love object with worldly gifts in order to obtain it. If all this is seen at such a gathering, it would be wise to stay silent.

Drinking parties

Men may drink in one another's houses and in bars and clubs, but should always do so moderately. Alcohol can very quickly distort the world and make weak men feel they are strong, and strong men believe they are weak. Drink only that which stimulates the mind and the fervor of the soul; that is, the best fruit, herb or vegetable juice taken, if possible, from the wild, and unfermented.

Outdoors

There are many diversions played out in the sunlight which stretch the mind and body, including walking, riding or climbing in unspoiled countryside, swimming in the sea, rivers and lakes and sailing or rowing upon the water. These are best enjoyed with company in a group or as a couple. Solitary diversions outside can also be of great comfort to the soul. Alone in a landscape the solitary man can often pierce the skin of the universe and speak to creation.

Other social diversions

Many indoor and outdoor sports and games are peculiar to a particular country and race. These may be learned with respect and enjoyed. A man should be selective, choosing only those diversions which suit his nature and which fulfill his temperament. Yet he should not be shy about attempting many of which he is ignorant, for only in the exploration of the world do we discover ourselves. Thus, a man should attempt much and choose little.

A citizen who discourses not entirely in his own language, nor wholly in the dialects of his own country, on various topics in the world, obtains great respect wherever he is.

Opposite: Racing on wet sand. A celebration of male vitality.

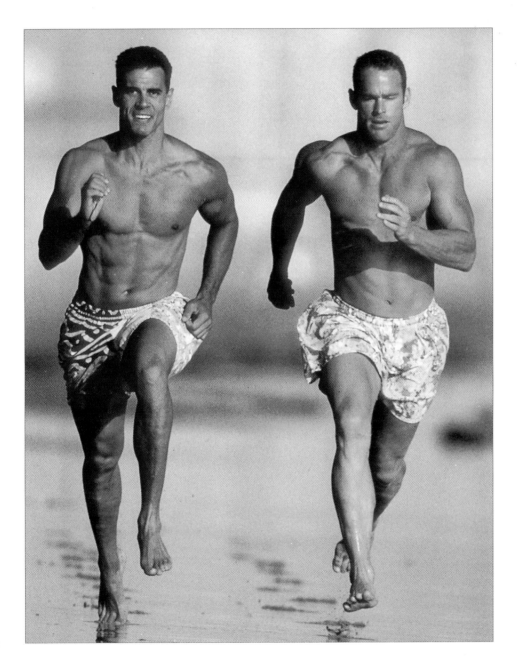

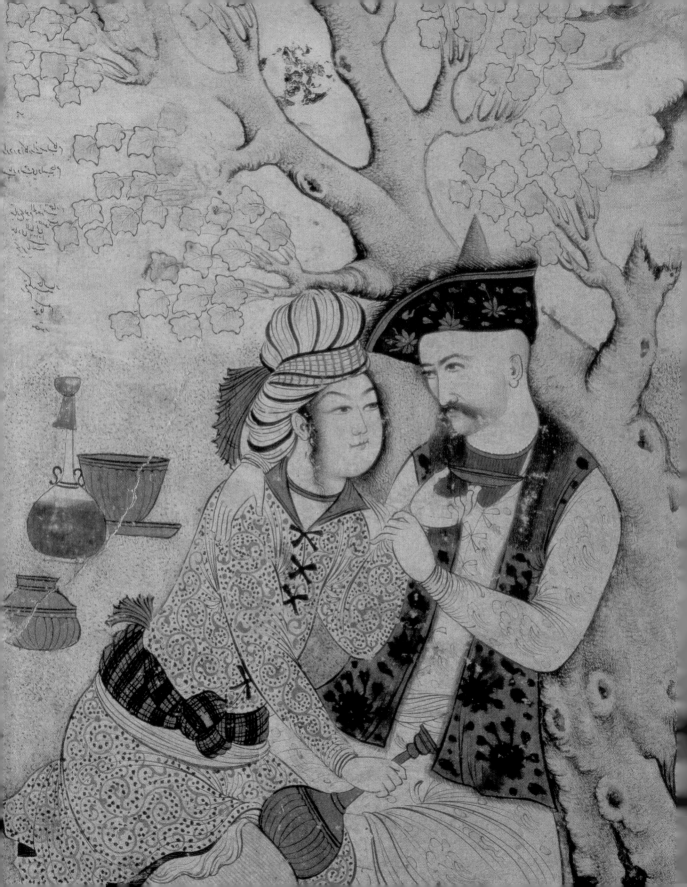

CHAPTER TWO
AMOROUS ADVANCES

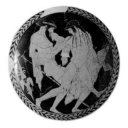

The first signs of sexual love are sight and sound. We may be instantly struck by another's beauty or by the sound of his voice. This sound has a timbre that touches us, drawing us to it as a magnet to iron. We long to be near, to inspect more closely, to fall in love more deeply. We long to touch, to see if this presence is real.

We may only catch a glimpse, a profile or a fleeting reflection in a mirror, or a shadow passing—yet we will know, for such glimpses are like daggers that drive deep into our soul. Then we are enslaved, walking like a ghost of ourselves, longing to be fed by yet another glimpse, so that we are destined to follow or wait in the shadows for that same sight. Be bold then and show yourself in all your radiance, because a love that is not a mutual passion is a sad, destructive force and should not be nurtured. Step forward out into the light and meet the one you desire. Do not flinch from that desire, for it is true.

Once your eyes have met you will know whether the interest is mutual. Desire cannot be disguised and is too powerful a force to be suppressed or hidden. Continue to be brave; if you can keep his gaze upon you by the passion of your own gaze, that is good. Walk toward him, drawing nearer yet all the while putting off the time when you will exchange your first words, for that sound will break the union of gaze which you have forged. You may merely issue an invitation, a request that he follow you, then you will turn and leave.

There are no rules to love. It is mysterious and can bloom

Opposite: A portrait of Shah Abbas I with one of his pages. A Persian miniature dated 1627.

Above: Zeus abducting Ganymede. The interior of a bowl painted by Pantasilea, 470 B.C.

39

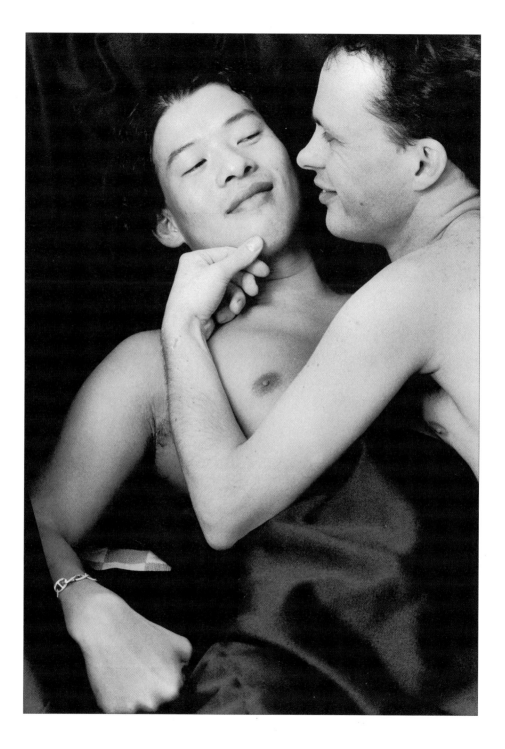

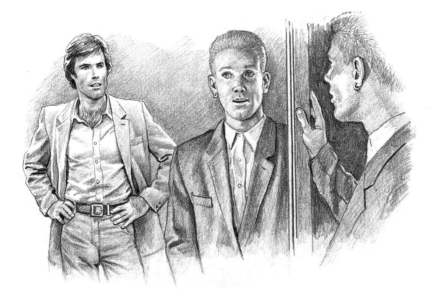

unexpectedly at the most inappropriate times, in the most unexpected places. Few clues will warn you of its arrival. Love may suddenly strike you in a relationship you had despised, or you may discover it in someone you thought you disliked. Love does not conform to age, race or gender.

ON TOUCHING

The first touch can be either a brush or a squeeze, or both of these.

Brushing is where the body lightly touches the other, glides and passes over. This is often done with the head looking away, as if the touching is quite accidental.

Squeezing is where the hand may take the arm of the other and give it a light squeeze, accompanied by a remark of friendship or praise. This is more intimate and may involve looking into each other's eyes for a moment and smiling. The hands may be lightly squeezed too and the forefinger may lightly brush the palm of the other's hand while you look into his eyes, smiling.

Touch is important, however slight. When first speaking with each

Opposite: Lovers. Contemporary society now throws together more people of different races than ever before. The lure of the dissimilar is a powerful aphrodisiac.

Above: A "fleeting reflection in a mirror." Immediate sexual attraction is one of the great mysteries of life.

other, lightly touch the desired one's fingers, or stroke the back of his hand. When it is acknowledged that such small gestures are freely received with delight and responded to, you may move on to more intimate touching.

The nape of the neck and the ear lobes are highly sensitive. Stroke the brow and the cheeks tenderly. Run your fingers lightly down the inside of the arm and with a rocking movement stroke the crook of the elbow. The base of the neck is another area that gives much pleasure.

If the courtship continues, touch forms part of the embrace and comes in three different kinds: rubbing, pressing and piercing. Rubbing may occur when two lovers are speaking freely with each other and walking slowly. One may embrace the other so that their bodies rub against each other, very slowly and gently, or the loins only may move, bucking slowly against the other's in gentle mimicry of the act of love.

Pressing is when one lover thrusts the other against a wall or pillar and embraces him with energy, pressing hard.

Piercing is where beneath the clothes the lover has an erection and presses it hard against his lover so that both can feel the hard shaft of the organ. One lover will then take the hand of the other and enclose

The Kiss. Gay affection can now be expressed in public, a change which has occurred only in the last fifteen years.

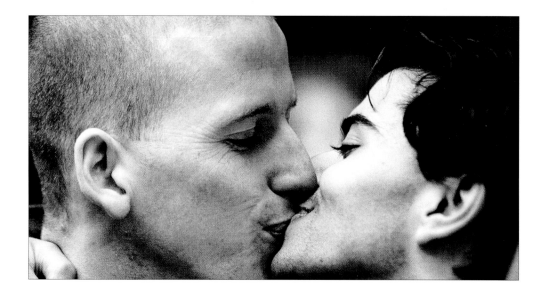

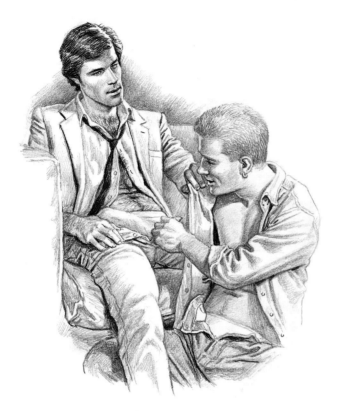

The powerful charge of gently undressing a new lover

it over the shaft. That is called cupping the stem.

Take time in undressing each other, for each button or fastener that is undone will reveal more flesh that may be coaxed into sensuality. Use your tongue upon the nipples. They will respond, however flat or small they might seem at first. Even a man who has been indifferent before will go mad with desire if his nipples are tenderly stroked, kissed, licked gently, then sucked.

Embraces come in many forms. There is the embrace of the thighs, when one man is seated upon the floor and the top half of the other is lying upon the bed, his feet touching the floor. In this position the thighs can be hugged and the inside of the thighs stroked, then licked gently.

The embrace of the *jaghana*—that part of the body from the navel to the thighs. This is when you collect and lift your lover, holding him firmly beneath by the buttocks and burying your face in his belly and covering his flesh with kisses. These moments might entail much scratching, biting or licking.

The embrace of the breasts. This is when the lovers press their breasts together after having stroked and licked the nipples, so that now the nipples are erect and they touch each other. By using swaying and careful delicate movements the nipples will continue to stimulate one another and drive you both to a frenzy of ecstasy.

The embrace of the forehead is when one lover touches the brow, eyelids or the nose of the other with his lips. The eyelids are especially sensitive and must be brushed with the utmost tenderness. This is often done after love-making and before sleep and will give the recipient a deep peaceful sleep full of dreams of happiness.

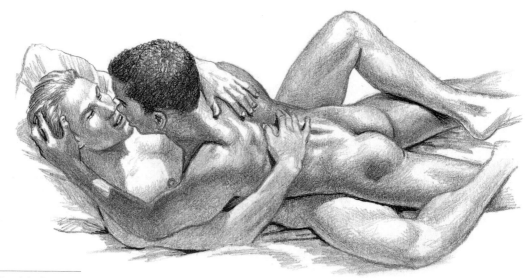

The Twining of the Creeper.

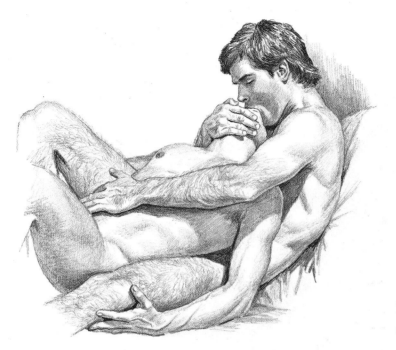

The Mixture of Sesame Seed
with Salt.

When in love there are four further embraces:

~ The twining of the creeper (*Jataveshtitaka*)
~ The climbing of the tree (*Vrikshadhirudhaka*)
~ The mixture of sesame seed with salt (*Tila-Tandulaka*)
~ The flower duet (*Kshiraniraka*)

When two lovers are closely entwined, their limbs entangled and one
has his head bent and the other is searching his eyes while their lips are
ready to kiss each other—this is called the twining of the creeper.

When a man places one foot upon the foot of the lover and his other
foot on one of the other's thighs, passes one of his arms round his lover's
back and the other upon his shoulders and seems to be in that posture of
climbing up his lover, that embrace is called the climbing of the tree.

When lovers lie on the floor or a sofa or bed and are entwined so closely that their arms and legs wrap around each other, this is called the mixture of sesame seed with salt.

When lovers embrace each other so hard amidst the act of penetration, not thinking of any pain or hurt, when all their limbs are entangled and they are singing with ecstasy, it is called the flower duet—because it is like the male flowers of the gourds opening very early in the morning and dipping their stamens, nestling close to each other.

CARESSING

The fingers are highly sensitive and merely a light touch on the beloved's body will give immense pleasure. Lie next to each other and let your hands hover above the other's body, merely brushing the hairs or lightly brushing the skin as if your fingers were a feather. Weave patterns with your fingertips over his stomach and around the genitals, but without touching them. Stroke his pubes and between his thighs. Let your fingers hover over the hairs upon his chest and nipples, brushing them a little, then breathe warm air upon his nipples.

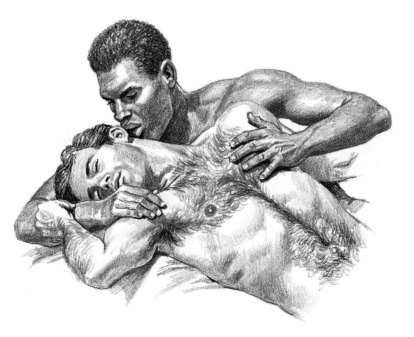

Caressing. The drowsy sensuality where all the nerves are heightened and lulled at the same time.

ON KISSING

Courtship involves many acts before complete sexual union. In order to taste the depths of sensual delights, do not hurry any of these phases. Relax fully into each one and let them find their own tempo.

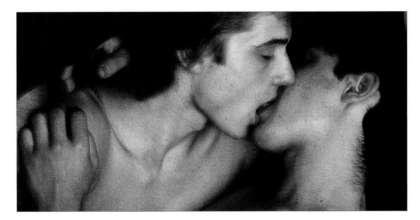

Kisses at the height of passion.

To kiss is one of the first ways of exploring the beloved. There are many types of kiss, from the most tender to the most passionate. Each one will bring you closer in your union, but on the first few meetings kissing, embracing, scratching and biting should all be done in moderation, if at all, and suitable pauses taken to rest and relax. Never ask the beloved whether particular behavior is to his liking. Such mannered enquiry is highly irritating, and shows lack of sensitivity. Lovers have no need to ask because all should be understood and known between them, especially matters of physical love-making.

To kiss each other's lips is the height of sensual ecstasy, but there are many other places for kissing: the brow, the eyelids, the throat, the ear lobes, the nape of the neck, the breasts, the nipples, the belly, between the thighs, in the cleft of the buttocks, the shoulder blades, the toes and feet. Kissing in these places is but the prologue to licking, for the tongue is ever-active in the kiss.

New lovers start cautiously without the tongue, and the first kiss is when the lips merely brush softly against each other. If the love is genuine, this act, barely touching, a mere brush of lip against lip, will hasten all sorts of unrest and longing.

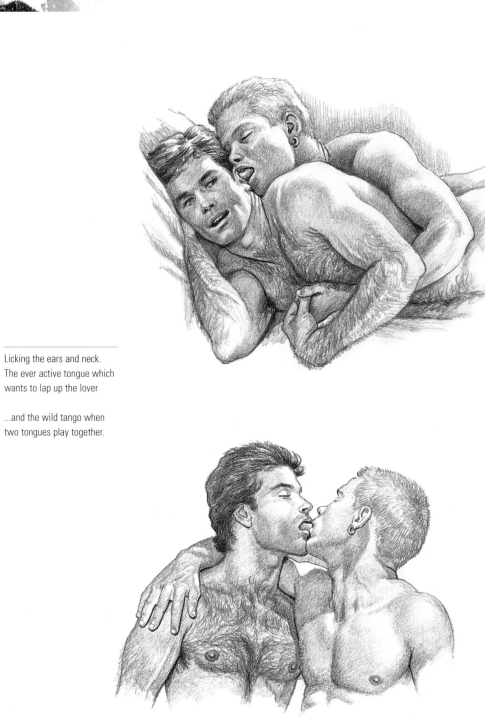

Licking the ears and neck.
The ever active tongue which
wants to lap up the lover

...and the wild tango when
two tongues play together.

The second kiss is when the lips are pressed hard against the lover's but the mouth is kept closed.

The third kiss is when such tender touching of the lips has begun as in the first kiss, but now the head is moved a little this way and that, so a motion starts, moistened by saliva. The eyes are closed while this occurs, and if in love a dream will be sure to start, a dream of paradise.

The fourth kiss is when the mouth is opened and the tongue enters the lover's mouth and moves to caress the inner lip. This can be done slowly, the tongue arching and probing at the same time.

The fifth kiss is when the tongue is moved energetically back and forth. The tongue is run over the sensitive surface of the gums to the top of the mouth, where the tip darts across the delicate membranes of the upper part of the mouth. Then the lover's tongue is sucked; this is called the soul kiss.

The sixth kiss is when the two tongues probe each other's mouths at the same time, both exploring the mouths of each other. This is often done at the height of passion and is called the bliss kiss.

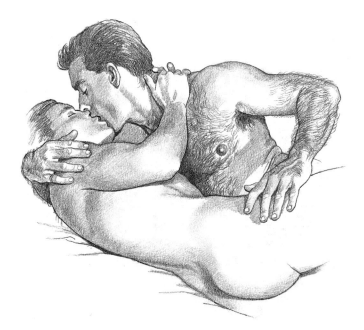

The bliss kiss, where the tongues anticipate mutual orgasm.

49

BITING AND SCRATCHING

Foreplay can often become rough when love is intense, but any pain is absorbed into the intensity of feeling. Both scratching and biting can be used in gentler love-making.

All parts of the body are suitable for biting, except for the upper lip, the tongue and the eyes. The forehead, lower lip, neck, cheeks, chest and nipples, the sides of the body, the armpits, thighs, knees, calves, feet and toes—all offer opportunities for this sensual love play. The sexual organs themselves can also be involved, though great care and tenderness must be used for these extra-sensitive parts of the body. When great delicacy is employed here, much pleasure can be gained.

There are times when the love experienced is so great that it feels as if one's rib cage will burst. Collecting the lover to you in a strong embrace and scratching him might be the only way to release the immensity of emotion. The nails draw a pattern upon the back, a signature of your passion, or the nails can incise a half moon. When the half moons are impressed opposite each other, they are called a circle. They will describe a pattern that remains for a moment or two and then fades.

Scratching which draws blood can also occur, generally at the height of passion (see the warnings on blood and the risk of infection, pages 66, 136). It can occur after an angry parting and form part of the love-making during reconciliation. These are times when guilt and anguish are expressed through love and small tokens of such pain seem to have value beyond themselves.

Sometimes scratching is used as a mark of being in love, with one man bearing the initials of his lover upon his breast or neck. When three marks with the nails are made close to one another near the nipple of the breast, it is called the swan. These marks are made before the beloved goes upon a journey and are there as his lover's signature.

The teeth are often used after kissing with tongues. Small gentle bites upon the lips, ear lobes, cheeks, breast, stomach and thighs may not leave even a small mark. Deeper kissing with the teeth pressed down hard and sucking in the flesh will leave an indentation called a love bite. There are many different bites.

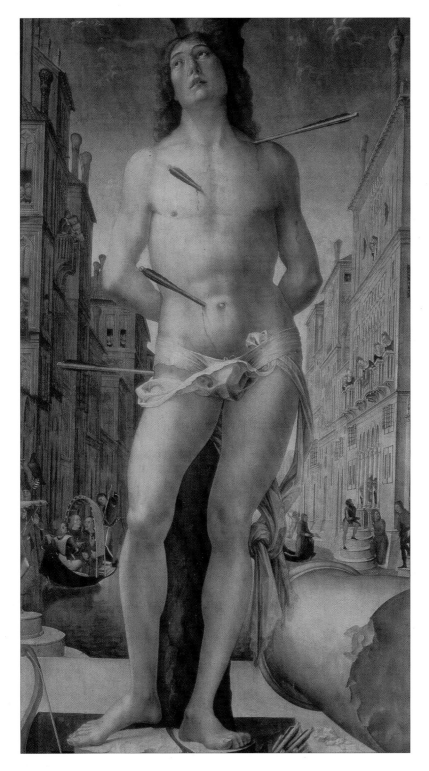

The Martyrdom of St. Sebastian, by Liberale da Verona (1445-1527). A favorite subject with Renaissance painters, which allowed them to glorify the sado-masochistic aspect of homoeroticism.

The Eight Love Bites:

> The hidden or discreet bite (*gudhaka*)
> The swollen or impressed bite (*ucchunaka*)
> The pointed bite (*bindu*)
> The necklace of points or dots (*Dindu-mala*)
> The coral jewel (*pravalamani*)
> The necklace of gems (*Manimala*)
> Scattered Clouds (*Khandabhraka*)
> The chewing of the wild boar (*varaha-charvita*)

The hidden or discreet bite is where the teeth are gently pressed on the lower lips so as to leave marks that do not last. A later and more interesting interpretation is that the bite is hidden from the public gaze and so is often made upon the buttocks. The skin is bitten and chewed almost angrily, leaving a small, round reddened patch of skin. Such bites can be arranged in patterns. A circular mark with one bite in the center and five around it is called the "camellia" because it resembles the flower.

The swollen or impressed bite can be similar to the first version of the discreet bite, but it is done more forcefully so that the mark stays red for longer. Here again there is another variation, when clusters of love bites are grouped together like a bouquet. This is sometimes called the "rose bite."

The impressed, pointed and coral jewel bites are made on the cheeks; kiss marks on the ear and scratch and bite marks on the cheeks are considered ornamental. Pointed marks occur when a small piece of skin is seized between the teeth and pulled, leaving small indentations of varying shape and color.

The coral jewel occurs when the same spot is squeezed several times with the lips and teeth. This results in a mark like a carnation flower.

When the coral jewel mark is made in a line or ring it is called a line of jewels. The necklace is where a ring of both impressed and pointed bites form a chain around the neck, or the upper arm, and perhaps even the thigh or waist.

Scattered clouds describes a number of small, pointed marks made in the same area, say on the breast, and different amounts of skin are seized and pulled for different lengths of time, so the shapes and colors are varied.

The chewing of the wild boar is when two necklaces are made around the thighs or stomach to frame the sexual organs. The nearer to the genitals the necklaces are, the more wild the boar is.

Only love play that increases passion should be engaged in first. Other amusements can be left until later in the relationship, when a greater variety can be enjoyed. Variety is necessary in love and can help produce still greater love. All acts of love play should be indulged in and enjoyed equally by the partners. If men act according to each other's liking, their love for each other will not be lessened even during the course of one hundred years.

BEATING WITH THE PRICK

When the penis is erect and much love-play is continuing, it is very satisfactory if one partner beats the body of the other with his hard prick. He holds it in his hand and bats it over the face of the lover, who tries to catch it with his mouth. The game is not to allow him to do so, and to continue beating his cheeks, nose and brow. The other place for this beating is the lover's buttocks, before penetration. When the buttocks are plumped up and ready, then is the time to bounce the erect penis off them, beating them hard so that your lover's flesh will flush pink. This is called "punishing love."

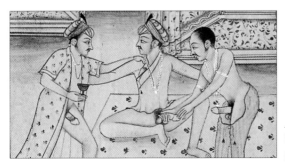

Modern Indian miniature painted in the Mughal style.

SIZE AND COMPATIBILITY

There is a mythology about the size of the male organ. This is not surprising given the history of veneration that the organ, the fount of life, has had. Art has often exaggerated and glorified its proportions, so it is not uncommon to find men anxious about the size of their penis. Such worries are best removed by speaking to others and by exhibiting

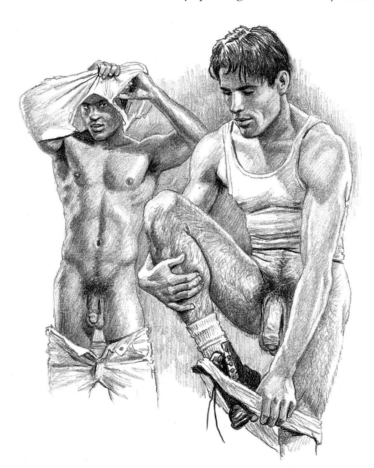

In the changing room, a good place for observing other men's attractiveness and differences in size

the organ, so that it can be viewed and its charms and qualities discussed. In love-making, it is not the size that matters but the skill with which the organ is used.

However, there are men who long to fellate large organs out of worship. They will obsessively search for the greatest organ, enslaving themselves and desiring only to possess it. A very large and noble penis is not always a happy accident for those so equipped. By virtue of this one physical attribute such men are too much in demand, and while their bodies are over-exercised their minds and souls are starved, with the result that their intellect and emotions are diminished.

Orifices, too, come in many sizes, for we are all individuals, and everything about us is as singular as our fingerprints. Though it is often said that orifices can expand to a much greater size, this is often not as easy to achieve as people and books claim. The perfect solution is to find lovers who complement each other in their physical shape and size. Where the anal orifice lies is vital to which position in love-making is used. In some men the space between the scrotum and the anus is small, while in others it is bigger.

The male organ, as we have observed, varies in shape, width and length. Some have large bulbous heads, while others are pointed; some are circumcized while others are not; some are curved while others are straight. Some organs will fit more naturally into the curve of the rectum, while others might well miss massaging the prostate gland, which is the seat of so much pleasure. Again the position will determine how the most exquisite pleasures are gained.

POSITIONS

There are four basic positions in which to make love: standing, kneeling, sitting and lying down. There are variations within these four positions, the most variations offering themselves in the last position. Positions which are happiest for the couple depend very much on comparative size and weight. If one partner is very large and the other small, then some positions may be awkward and well-nigh impossible. Your physical characteristics as well as your particular desires will determine which position you prefer. Often pieces of furniture, chairs and stools will be useful to help give support and thrust. Old-fashioned bedsteads serve a purpose as the brass or iron railings and supports are useful for providing added thrust and tension. Be adventurous: try them all to see which suit you.

STANDING

The standing positions are athletic and have great aesthetic beauty. Their erotic power can be enhanced by the use of mirrors.

1. Two-Pillar Position. This is only possible with two men whose loins are on the same level. If there is a disparity in loin height, then the penetrated partner is lifted up and on the other, his ankles twining around the other's calves and then resting his feet upon a step to give both leverage and height. In this position, it is not easy to kiss.

2. A variation is when the penetrator stands and his partner bends over a bed or chair. Once penetrated the upper part of the partner bending is pulled back in a close embrace, while his neck and ear is nibbled and bitten.

3. The Pillar and the Ivy. In this position the lovers are facing each other, and the one who is penetrated climbs and twines his legs around the other's thigh. With this position it is obviously better if the one that climbs is much smaller and lighter than the one that penetrates. The lover standing can then push and pull the other while they kiss.

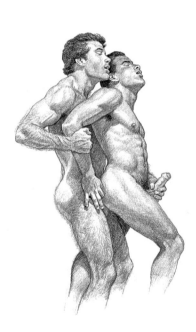

The Two Pillar Position.

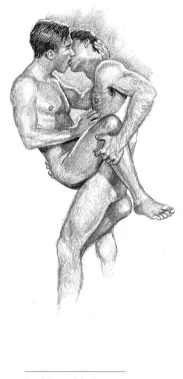

The Pillar and the Ivy.

KNEELING

1. The man who penetrates kneels and pulls his partner upon him, so that the partner straddles him like a butterfly poised above a flower. The butterfly is in control, timing the strokes, supported by his hands and feet, while the kneeling partner supports himself behind with his hands. A good kissing position if the butterfly, held in position by his legs, now embraces his lover and kisses him.

2. The lover kneeling is now in control. He grips his lover by the hips and buttocks and moves him up and down while supporting himself with his hands upon his lover's knees.

3. The Two-Dog Position. The lover who is penetrated is upon his hands and knees, the other kneels behind him. This is a popular and common position, because the penetrator can move very swiftly and therefore heighten the excitement, but it makes kissing very difficult.

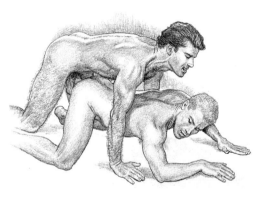

The Two-Dog Position.

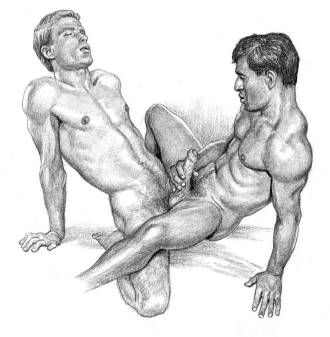

The Kneeling Butterfly Position.

57

SITTING

1. The penetrator can sit upon a chair without arms and his lover can sit astride him and support himself with his feet or toes upon the floor. For extra support it is best to have the back of the chair against or near a wall.

2. If the penetrator lies on his back over a stool, allowing his head and shoulders to touch the floor on one side and his feet the other, his erection then is seen in the most noble and piercing position. The lover can sit astride him, turning any way he likes and controlling his movements and the pleasure he gives to his partner. He can support himself with his hands upon the side of the stool.

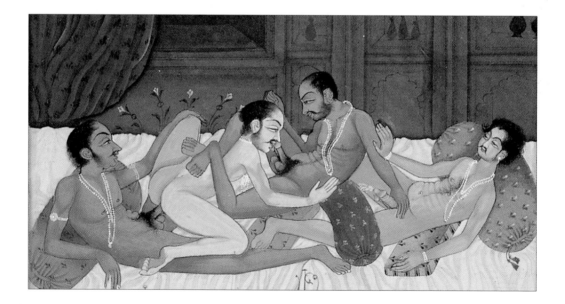

Permutations of pleasure.
Modern Indian miniature.

Here the passive lover almost becomes the active one in controlling the timing of the strokes.

Another variation, where a hard surface gives greater leverage.

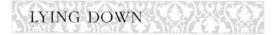

LYING DOWN

Some people prefer making love lying down on a hard surface like the floor or the ground outside rather than a bed or sofa. The most ecstatic sex may be had on a hard, sandy beach. Whatever the place of our choosing, the positions—and there are many of them—remain the same.

1. The Clasping Position. The penetrated lies on his stomach, his buttocks raised and supported by a pillow placed under them. The penetrator lies on top and stretches himself out over the length of

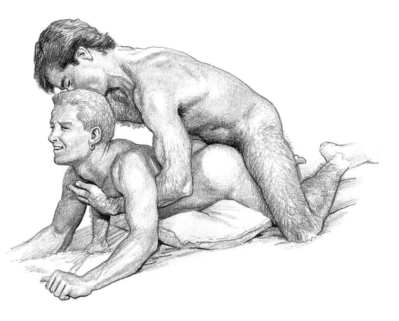

The Clasping Position, where the penetrator should show consideration and take care not to become too aggressive.

his lover's body. The drawbacks of this position are that kissing is difficult and that the member of the man being penetrated may become buried in the pillows or bedclothes and cannot be massaged into orgasm by either lover. Once penetration has been achieved and you are in happy congress, it might be a good idea to change the position, perhaps by turning your bodies sideways. However, some couples may prefer the original position, but swap-

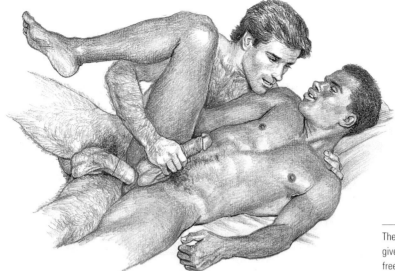

The Sideways Position; this gives the penetrated more freedom to move and control the strokes.

ping over once the penetrator has achieved orgasm so that he in turn may be penetrated. In this scenario the partner initially penetrated will not want to stimulate his organ before he gains entry. This arrangement can work marvelously well: both partners will be so intensely stimulated that their love-making will continue quite smoothly into another session.

2. Sideways Position. Once entry is gained in this position the penetrator can massage the organ of his lover, bringing him to orgasm at the same time. When the legs are also entwined, this is called the "pressing position."

3. On Top. This is a better position for kissing. The penetrator lies beneath his lover who lies across him with his knees bent. A variation on this is where the two lovers lie feet to head and gain leverage by holding each other's calves.

4. The Crab Position. A continuation of position 3, this is sometimes difficult to achieve. The lover gains entry while he and his partner are lying head to toe on the floor. Then simultaneously they raise their bodies, supporting themselves on their arms and legs. This position stimulates the prostate more effectively than any other, though you will find the thrusts are more difficult because your partner will be almost floating above you.

5. Face-to-face: The Yawning Position. The penetrated lies on his back, his thighs open, knees bent and his loins thrust upwards by a pillow or cushion. This position is good for kissing and for massage of his organ.

6. The Rising Position. The same position as 5, but now the penetrated lifts his legs higher and rests them over his lover's shoulders.

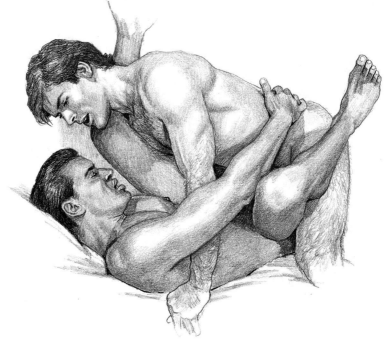

The Half-Rising Position, where the penetrated feels that he can almost engorge his partner.

7. The Half-Rising Position. It begins as the same position as 6, but only one leg is thrown over the lover's shoulder; the other leg is bent around the lover's thighs.

8. The Pressed Position. In this face-to-face position the penetrated bends his legs and draws them up until his knees touch his chin.

9. The Half-pressed Position. When only one leg is bent upwards and the other stretches out.

ON PENETRATION

An enema should be taken an hour before sexual congress. Once all waste matter is voided, the anus should be gently washed, not only outside but the inner lining, too. Choose scented soaps which turn your lover on. After it has been washed, the anus can be oiled, as well as the space between the scrotum and anus, the crack between the buns, and the testicles and penis. The anus is lined with particularly sensitive nerve endings which will respond immediately when touched, sending all kinds of pleasurable messages to the brain. So feel no shame about your use of this orifice for sexual pleasure. It was ordained so.

If you are inexperienced in sexual love, it is best to spend a little time getting to know the secret parts of yourself and how they work. Also spend some time in looking after them. After voiding, wash the anal opening with care. Examine it by laying a mirror flat on the floor or a chair and straddling yourself over it. Practice controlling the sphincter muscle, drawing it in and letting it out. Then, using a lubricant on your finger, explore inside, deeper and deeper.

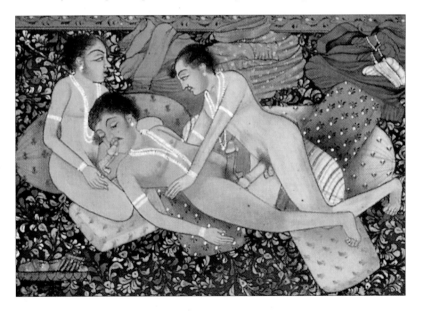

Homoerotic scene. Modern Indian miniature.

(Ensure that your nails are cut very short, with no abrasive edges. It is wise to check the nails of your lover, too. The interior membrane of the rectum can be torn, which may lead to serious infection.) If you move two or three fingers in and out you will discover that, once the sphincter muscle is relaxed, there is no pain associated with this movement. You will also see how much larger the anal opening can grow once it is relaxed and is familiar with the touch of your fingers.

Remember that pain is caused by fear and apprehension; fear will tighten all the muscles in your body and make it unattractive to touch or fondle. Penetration should not be attempted if you and your partner are not completely relaxed and loving towards each other. Anything else is rape.

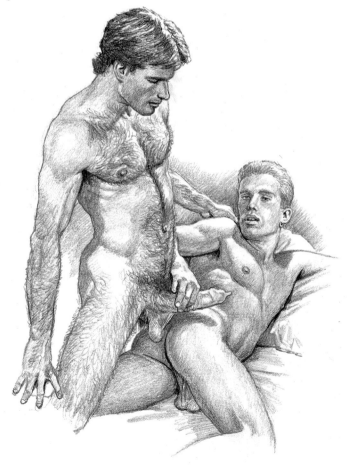

Putting on a condom, now an essential part of making love, can itself be an erotic act.

After much kissing, stroking and fondling, when you have licked and massaged each other, you can both then begin to explore the anal organ with your fingers, tongue and lips (see the note on washing above and the section on fellatio and rimming, page 68). Help your lover put on the condom and lubricate it thoroughly. Let him rest his organ in the cleft of your buttocks, rubbing it up and down and over the anal opening. Encourage him then to stop at the opening and press a little, then help him by guiding his organ into the opening. Let him get the head in and then pause and rest. Get used to this new feeling. Move your loins back and forth a little so that you can control the pace, then allow him to push a little more, pause again and so on, several times if you wish, until your lover has thrust his whole length in.

Do not rush; try to hold back. The best lovers are those with the greatest control over their timing of orgasm. The longer a man stays inside his lover the greater the pleasure for both. Now is the time to change position but without withdrawing completely. You can ask which new position is best for your lover, but while some lovers are reassured by loving words, others might find them an irritant and that they cause them to lose concentration. Discussion of the act and how to improve it should take place afterwards.

When inside, he can massage your organ with his hands. Sometimes the sensation inside the anus is so great that your spermatic orgasm will come later, for there is another orgasm, an interior one, that you will experience. This is because the prostate gland is being massaged, and this gives a long glowing climax, quite different from the usual one. Tell your lover afterwards the position that gives you the greatest pleasure in this respect.

SAFE SEX

If you are a couple of some years' standing who are loyal to each other, who know and trust each other, then there is no need to use condoms in penetrative sex. This is a decision which you as a couple must take. If either of you expresses doubt or fear about unprotected sex, it is best to be scrupulous about safety. You would also be wise to have a yearly test for HIV.

If you change partners and start playing the scene, or even have the occasional romantic liaison with others, it is always essential to use condoms when engaging in penetrative sex.

For some, this is the ultimate act of sexual congress. To be inside a lover's body, and for him to be inside you, is a mystical as well as a physical union. It should always be a loving act which occurs after much preliminary love play. Only in this way will your bodies be receptive and pliable. If you are both new lovers and new to each other, let this act be a late development to look forward to as you build your relationship, so that it is the final flowering of all your prior sexual love-making.

Remember, too, not to withdraw too quickly after orgasm; it is best to stay inside and withdraw very slowly and carefully some minutes afterwards. You must each give time to the other to descend slowly from the peaks you have reached. Do not wait too long, however, as the condom is more likely to slip off when the erection has waned.

The rectum is a high risk area for HIV infection and Hepatitis B, because it is made up of a mucous membrane which absorbs liquids. (It is well worth having an injection against Hepatitis B.) Ensure that you use only extra strong condoms and with them a water-based lubricant like KY; with oil-based lubricants the immense friction can disintegrate the condoms. Saliva as a lubricant for penetration is not much use because it dries out very quickly.

Can the HIV virus be caught in the act of oral sex? As the virus lives in the semen and in blood, it would seem that swallowing the semen is a sure-fire way of catching it. But there has never been any proven link between fellatio and the infection. Be cautious. Never permit a penis in your mouth if you have bleeding gums or a mouth ulcer. The lining of the mouth is quite different from that of the rectum; it is much more difficult for the virus to infect you through the mouth, for the saliva has enzymes which destroy bacteria. Keep your mouth, gums and teeth in good health by regular dental visits. The most sensible course is not to swallow the semen. If any semen does go into the mouth, spit it out. Fellatio is thought to be only a minimal risk activity, so take heart. Try using the technique *sangara* below, in which no semen flow is emitted in orgasm.

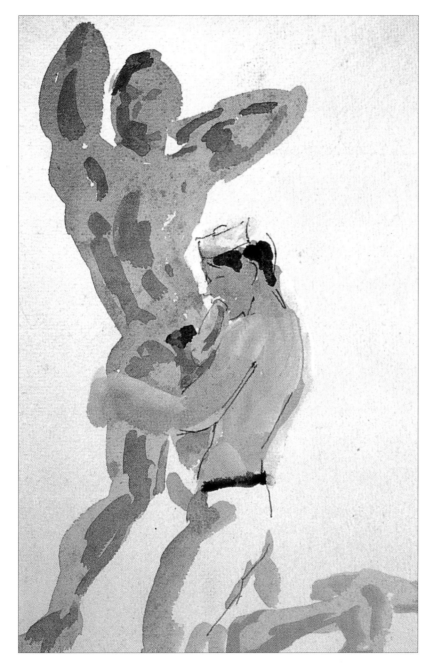

Sailor Fellating a Nude, a watercolor by Duncan Grant (1885-1978). The muscular black man poses and gains more excitement from his reflection in an unseen mirror.

67

SUPERIOR COITION OR FELLATIO (*Auparishtaka*)

The Kama Sutra calls fellatio "superior" because the "third sex" performs in the mouth the act that takes place between the thighs during straight sex. The penis can be taken into the mouth when it is flaccid, then it can be licked and sucked very gently. It gives great pleasure to the fellator to have the penis slowly swell in the mouth until it becomes quite rigid. When the penis is flaccid the balls, too, can be taken into the mouth. The fellator can then embrace each of the three with his tongue, drop out two while he plays with one, or leave out the penis while he chews gently upon the balls and nibbles the scrotum. This is called "Eating Lunch."

When the penis is rigid there are six ways of fellatio.

1. The casual (*nimitta*). Holding the penis with one hand, placing the lips round the mast of the penis and licking the shaft up and down. This is a good beginning to excite your lover.

2. Nibbling the sides (*parshvatodasha*). The same as 1, except that as well as licking, allow the teeth as well as the lips to gently touch the shaft so that is kissed and sweetly bitten.

3. Internal pinching (*antah-sanddamsha*). Following on from above, allow the penis to enter the mouth

"Eating Lunch." The delights of extending the pleasure for both partners.

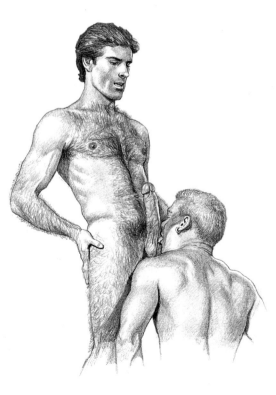

and suck while kissing. Hold the penis with one hand to guide it into the mouth. With the other hand, use your forefinger to enter the anal orifice and massage it gently.

4. Kissing and browsing (*chumbitaka* and *parimrishtaka*). Work upon the tip of the penis, kissing and licking around the rim of the head and with your tongue titillate the opening.

5. Sucking the mango (*amrachishitaka*). With the erect penis in your mouth, massage the shaft while sucking upon the head. Use your other hand to massage the highly sensitive area between the anus and the base of the penis.

6. Devouring (*sangara*). Do all of the above and suck with increasing force. When you feel that the lover is about to ejaculate, clench the hand into a tight fist and press hard just beneath the base of the cock. This will stop the flow of semen to the head of the penis, while allowing the man to experience a greater intensity of orgasm which will continue for much longer than if he emits in the usual manner.

The fellator can also fill his mouth with hot or cold water. He can bathe the penis in honey, cream or caviar; both partners will enjoy his licking it off. The important thing is to feel free and have fun.

Chewing chilies is common practice among heterosexuals—but why let them have all the enjoyment? However, use extreme caution when doing this, because the *glans penis* is exceptional-

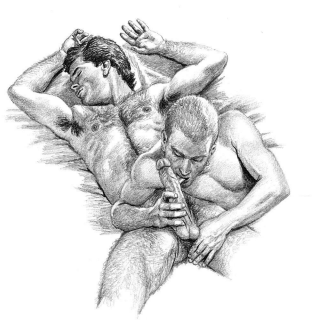

The beginning of the Casual, where the tongue very softly moves up and down the shaft.

Sucking the Mango. The more you practice the deeper you can take the shaft without gagging, and the more pleasure both will gain.

ly sensitive. First of all, choose your chili with care. Avoid the very hot ones, like scotch bonnets or Habanero (*Capsicum sinense*). Choose a Poblano, a Jalapeño or a Cascabel and poach it for about ten minutes in water. This gets rid of much of the pith, the hottest part. Leave to cool. Then start by nibbling the end which is the less hot part and work your way up. Stop when your mouth feels too hot. Capsaicin, which chilies contain, triggers the release of endorphins, the body's natural painkillers, and creates a sense of general well-being. So your pleasure is heightened already. Now your mouth is ready for the blow job. If you both do it at the same time, you can enjoy the most ecstatic sixty-nine you'll ever have. If your cock hurts too much, dip it into cold water and keep a cold sponge on it.

ORGIES

The Kama Sutra celebrated the highly erotic potential of orgies. Sadly, in some countries today, they are illegal. Before the AIDS era there was a great vogue for private orgies in the States. Some men gave weekly sessions and invited the boys from the nearest gay bar, often greeting them at the door almost naked to make clear the nature of the gathering.

People congregating together are often shy and inhibited, and fall back on social conventions, drinking and chatting, so it is important for one man to strip off and begin the action. Once an orgy is under way, anything goes. One man can fellate another and masturbate a third, while himself being penetrated. Generally it begins with men pairing off, but very soon someone else will want to join in the action. At most orgies it is decreed that any flesh going is available to everyone present, that all men are welcome to be naked and lustful, that youth and beauty must be shared equally, that genuine desire is the most beautiful of all emotions when it is seen in uninhibited action.

A man who is free in the knowledge that sexual pleasure and display are his to enjoy can multiply all types of sexual congress, imitating the different ways of the birds and the beasts. These various

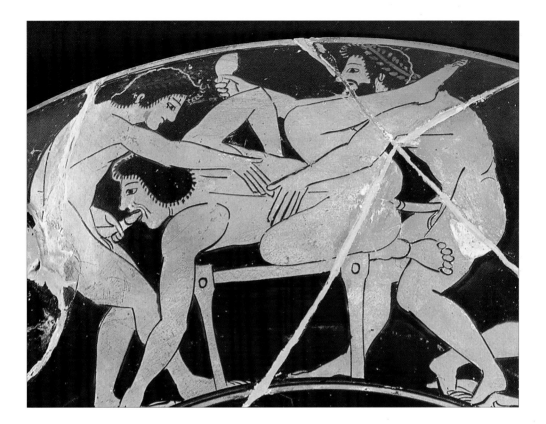

kinds of congress, performed according to the custom of each country, and the liking of each individual, generate love, respect, and friendship in the hearts of men.

Scene on a Greek wine cup, showing a threesome, attributed to the Pedieus painter, sixth century B.C.

ON THE DIFFERENT KINDS OF SEXUAL LOVE

When two men who have been in love for some time still insist on coming together despite obstacles or hazards not of their own making, it is called "the brave congress."

When one of a pair of lovers returns after a long, anguished parting, each needing the other as part of his necessary self, then their love-making is called "the fused as one congress."

When lovers are reconciled after a quarrel, when much bitterness and tears have been shed but their loving has triumphed, then their love-making is called "the triumphant congress."

When two men come together in the first flush of their love, while their love for each other is still in its infancy, theirs is called the "congress of subsequent love."

When a man makes love to himself by exciting himself into orgasm by any means available, it is called "the hopeful congress." There are many variations in which men make love to themselves. When a man is sad and lonely, it is called "the comfort congress." Or when a man is in despair and thinks himself unloved and ugly it is called "the congress of misfortune." Or when a man is old and tired it is called "the congress of nostalgia." When two men come together though they are both attached to different loves, their sexual meeting is called "the congress of artificial love."

When a man makes love to one man while thinking of another, it is called "the congress of transferred love."

The sexuality that takes place between two men who are genuinely attached to one another is called "spontaneous congress."

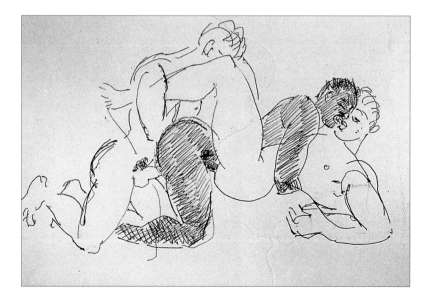

Pas de Trois 3, a drawing by Duncan Grant. The synchronization of the thrusts is essential.

ON ARTIFICIAL QUARRELS

Some men have a love of the theater and want to act out their own personal dramas in their love lives. These men are adept at creating quarrels, which may be works of art in themselves. Such men tend to put their nearest and dearest through much hell in order to fulfill themselves. They are happiest in the midst of tirades which typically have come from nowhere. They will pick up on a small detail and enlarge it out of all proportion. They may be sobbing and seemingly in great pain and misery, but these men are in fact fulfilling a need. They are locked into a cycle of quarrel and reconciliation, which very often reflects behavior seen in one of their parents. It is more likely to have been the mother, who may have received the love she craved only after a quarrel. In adulthood the man will perpetuate this pattern by picking a quarrel in order to receive love.

The answer lies in making the man see the roots of his problem. Only when he understands why he is driven into committing this particular cycle of behavior can he stop. Friends or a professional counselor can help.

ON JEALOUSY

Jealousy is the most common reason for lovers' quarrels. Jealousy may be behind the behavior of the false quarrel, but then there is generally very little reason for it. Jealousy stems from people who feel insecure in their loving. Their insecurity has nothing to do with their partner, whose reaction may be to become more considerate and more passionate, all to no avail.

If a man feels unloved, he is probably out of love with himself. He secretly despises himself, or has no faith in himself, or feels he is unlovable because he has great flaws and failings. He fears that his partner is looking around for a perfect or more attractive man.

A man's early environment, if it failed to give him loving support, may be the cause. If surrounded by people or a person who was always over-critical, he may have learned at an early age to feel inadequate and completely at a loss.

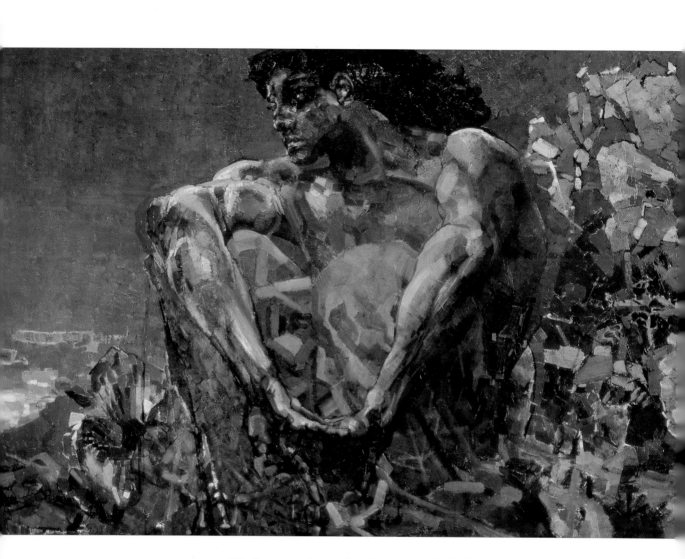

A brooding study of a young man by the Russian painter Mikhail Vrubel (1856-1910).

The best solution is for the man to look back into his childhood and to recognize how inadequate those adults were. He should feel within himself outrage that they could have treated a child with such lack of love and respect. This would be the first step towards gaining his own self respect. Sometimes a man needs professional help to reconcile himself with his childhood.

ON REAL QUARRELS

True love flowers with mutual respect, loving concern, and an understanding of a partner's need for his own private space. Each individual should possess space of his own. Though there will always be some differences of opinion in a love relationship, and they may well lead to quarrels, these differences exhibit the good health of the relationship.

One of the most important qualities in a loving relationship is a sense of humor. If two partners make each other laugh, then the relationship has a much greater chance of lasting. Quarrels are usually easily ended by making the other person laugh, or when both see the absurdity of the situation. All of us have bad moods, or days when nothing goes right. Our partners are there to suffer the testiness which is naturally fermenting within us.

However, there may be real quarrels over matters of deeply held principle. When these occur it is important to attempt to understand the other man's point of view, to eliminate the emotional aspect from the subject and to look at it coolly and rationally. The private space you have given each other should allow a difference of opinion. Try to agree to disagree and remain lovers. This is not as hard as it might seem. Lovers who stay together often discover in time that they have become closer as a result of their disagreement.

Some quarrels are so serious that they will drive a wedge between lovers. The disagreement may revolve around a person, whom one partner dislikes and with whom the other is obsessed. In such a case let obsession take its course. Then take a long look at the relationship to see whether or not the partners consider it worth saving. Such momentous decisions must not be made quickly; they should be discussed in detail over a period of time. Once a decision is made, though, it is best to act quickly upon it.

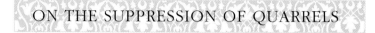

ON THE SUPPRESSION OF QUARRELS

In some relationships exists a fear of quarrels. The partners are so determined to make their relationship work and provide a happy context for each other that constant petty annoyances and the friction of living together are suppressed. If this suppression has lasted many years the partners will find themselves tired and distressed, with constant feelings of being unable to cope. Their love for each other will have become jaded and without sparkle. They may know that they still love each other but cannot dredge up much enthusiasm for the relationship.

The answer lies in telling the truth. Each partner should own up to having any disloyal thoughts about the other and confess them. Only by exploring these negatives can we be honest in our daily lives.

Sometimes, only one partner has suppressed the urge to quarrel. He will feel that his identity has been consumed by his blissfully unaware partner, to whom he has become an appendage. This is merely because he has refused to stand up for himself. The answer lies in stopping the suppression immediately.

In all these instances quarrels can be beneficial.

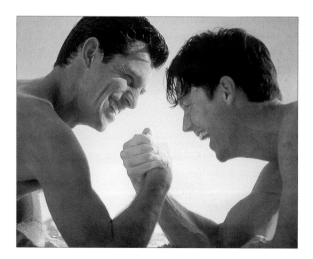

Right: Trial of strength.

Opposite: Out and about in New York. The beginning of social change as gay men openly show their affection.

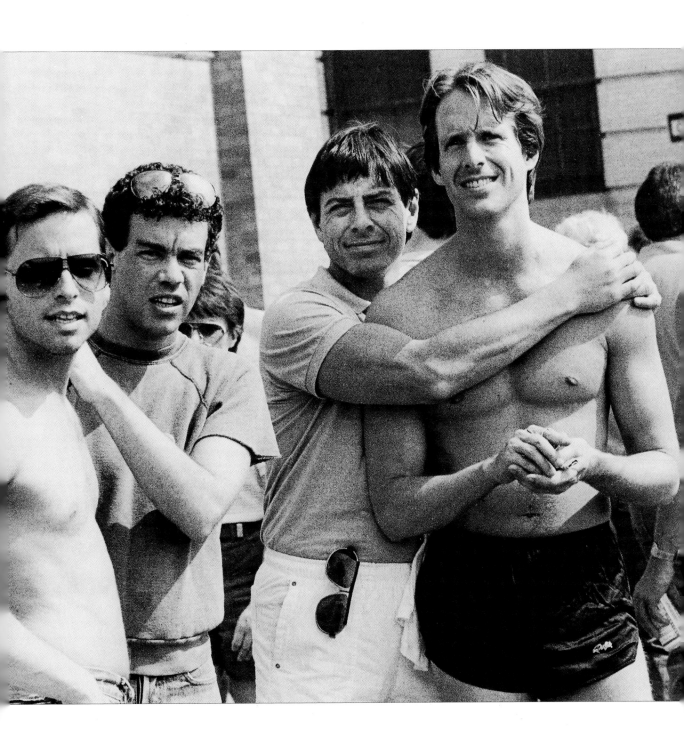

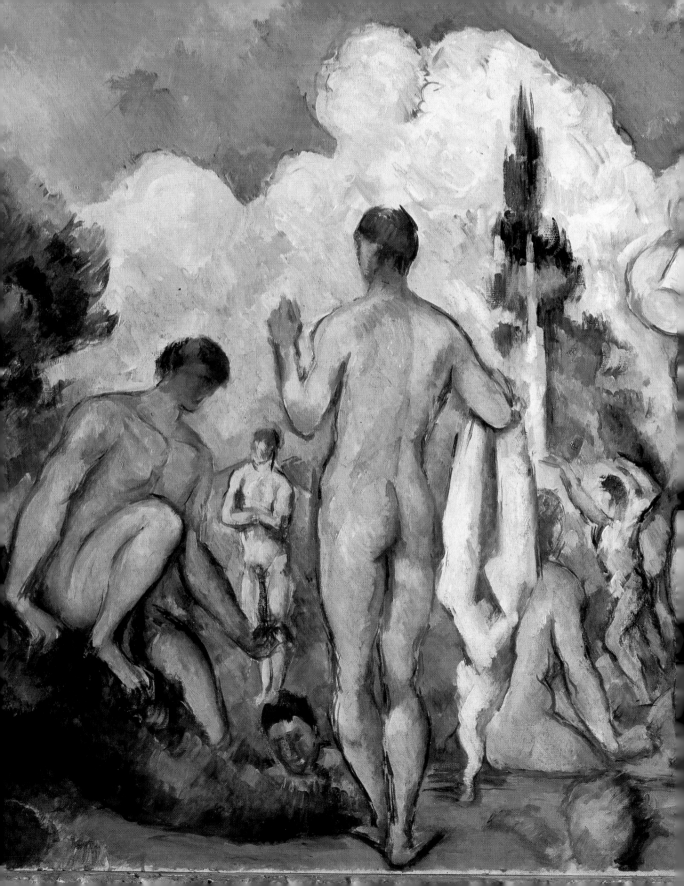

CHAPTER THREE:
MALE SEXUALITY AND SOCIETY

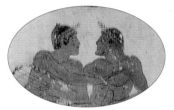

Male-dominated societies have been with us for many thousands of years. Inevitably they have also been phallocentric societies, in which the phallus is king and men can envisage no sexuality without it. In male-dominated societies women are often treated as second-class citizens, whose main purpose is to give birth and to nurture the young. Subordination of women allows the sexuality of males to become synonymous with dominion and aggression. The traditional structure of society, embodied in our culture, puts the male at the head of the household; he is the sole decision maker and the one who penetrates the female according to his will. In our society even fertilization is seen through a male perspective. Without semen, man's vital component, the human species would come to an end.

This misogynist view of the world is quite recent in man's eight-million-year-old life span. Early society was matriarchal. If we imagine *Homo sapiens* as an eighty-year-old man, then the age of matriarchy (*c.* 30,000—15,000 B.C.) would have occurred in the last hour of his life. We see it appearing in the ancient world certainly, but evidence suggests that matriarchal societies existed in prehistory. Throughout history Gnostic sects practiced equality of gender and celebrated homosexuality. (In these sects spiritual knowledge was attained directly and did not require the priest as intermediary.)

Opposite: Detail from *The Bathers,* by Paul Cézanne (1839-1906).

Above: Lovers at a banquet. From a fifth-century B.C Greek mural at Posidonia (Paestum), southern Italy.

This history places our present idea of masculinity in perspective. We know that throughout time there have been concepts of masculinity that the average straight male today would find difficult to accept. For example, in the ancient world and up until the late seventeenth century, males were expected to be bisexual. Social forces shape sexual ideals, which most people struggle to conform to because they want to appear 'normal.' But 'normality' is only the social construct of a particular time and place, and has no absolute or timeless authority. That is why the Bible, although a massive anthropological work of information, cannot be used to dictate moral standards to societies living two thousand years after it was written. Morality changes and grows as society re-evaluates its standards of right and wrong. After all, slavery was abolished less than two hundred years ago.

We must be grateful that in all societies certain people reject the idea of 'normal,' and question the authority of the orthodox majority . They want only to be true to themselves. They may be called renegades and heretics, and suffer persecution and punishment. We think of them as martyrs to the truth.

Clearly our view of male and female sexuality is undergoing a change. Feminists, intellectuals, and the gay community are challenging yesterday's notion of male sexuality as dominating and aggressive. Yet we have to cope with the fact that society's machinery is still running on these principles. Our laws and institutions, supported by the subliminal manipulating power of advertising, buttress a social framework whose maxims are that the straight male is boss, and that his is the only path leading to success and happiness.

Yet human nature, or male sexuality, does not change in a few thousand years. Male sexuality today is in a confused and unhappy state, unsure where it is, where it is going and what threatens it. Today's 'straight' male is often a puzzled creature.

Many straight men who acknowledge today's redefinition of gender still feel threatened by the rise of feminism and women's equality. They also know that they must not, because of social shame, give in to any gay desires that they might nurture. What is the truth about male sexuality?

In *The Kama Sutra* we have a graphic picture of the male as a pleasure-seeking prince, where women are like musical instruments for him to play upon. His view of sexuality is that any sexual act upon any part of the body that gives pleasure to both lovers is right and normal. Women are not shamed and humiliated just to increase his delight. They are, however, second fiddles in what is very much a male-orientated society.

We know from observing ourselves and from knowledge of the past that men are able to enjoy all kinds of sexual experience. Today's picture of the straight dominant male is a grave distortion of natural male sexual expression, and one which hides his many-faceted desire.

The straight male, confined completely by heterosexual norms, able only to desire one gender, is a very recent appearance, dating back to around 1700. Men were not previously thought of in such a limited way. The gay male today is much closer in his thinking and way of life to the historical male and should be proud of the connection. The heterosexual male may not wish to acknowledge this shared sexual past, but in remembering it the gay man will enrich his sexual nature and confirm his worth.

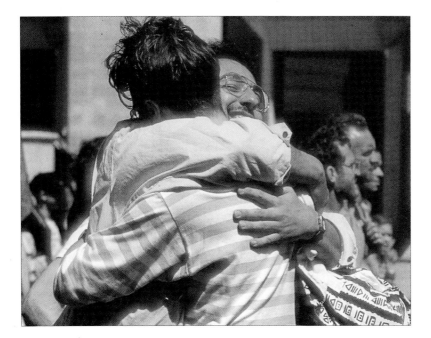

Gay Pride, London, 1990.

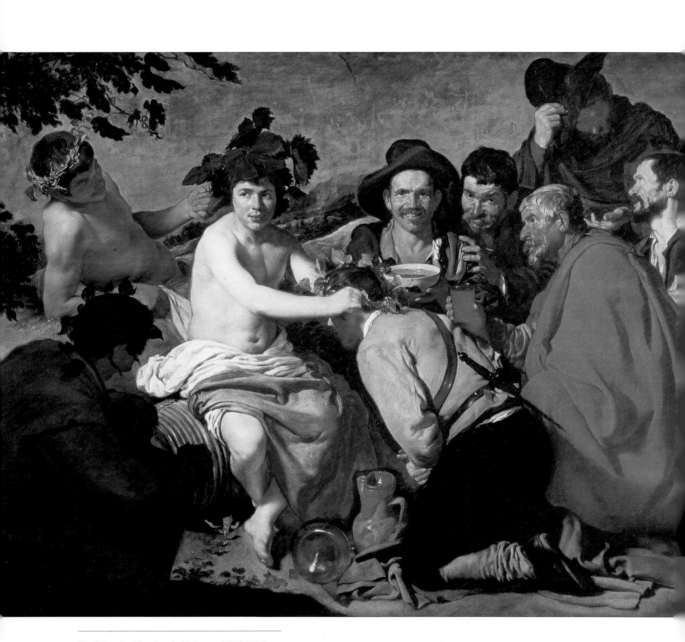

The Triumph of Bacchus, by Velásquez (1599-1660).
The pagan god of wine and sexual pleasure is adored
by devoted peasants, as if they are showing gratitude
for the best things in their lives.

82

THE BIOLOGY

It helps to understand our sexuality if we take note of our bodies' sexual responses. During the first of four stages of sexual readiness, we get excited, the heart rate and blood pressure increase, our breathing becomes heavier, the scrotum thickens, the testicles move upwards and we get an erection. The second stage, called the plateau, is where the erection is at its maximum size and a clear lubricating fluid, an alkaline secretion from the Cowper's gland, beads the head of the penis.

The third stage is the orgasm, where rhythmic contractions of the muscles at the base of the penis and of the urethral canal occur, ending in anything from three to seven spurts of seminal fluid at 0.8 second intervals. The fourth stage is the resolution, during which the body slowly returns to its normal state. Blood pressure, heart beat, and respiration reduce their rate, the testicles descend and the penis gradually becomes flaccid.

A healthy attitude toward sexuality depends very much upon the amount and accuracy of the information about sex obtained during childhood and adolescence. If we are given all the facts, no matter how shocking they might seem to some people, we can make an informed choice. However, sexual arousal and orgasm do not encompass the whole sexual experience: our physical reactions are heightened when our emotions and minds are involved.

CIRCUMCISION

This practice of cutting away some or all of the foreskin on the penis began with the ancient Egyptians, who operated on youths *en masse*. (There may be a practical reason for it beginning in Egypt. British soldiers in World War II who were uncircumcised suffered agonies from sand trapped beneath the foreskin.) Circumcision was practised by the Hebrews, for whom it became a religious rite. In practical terms circumcision may have some small hygienic advantage, although the foreskin is there to protect the *glans penis*. Uncircumcised men, however, are often said to have more sensitive penises than the circumcised.

Though the debate over circumcision persists, there seems to be no good reason for it to be done. The operation can be highly painful, it is often performed by people not adequately trained, and the area can sometimes become infected. Recently the practice has been attacked as a form of child sexual abuse sanctioned by religion and state. The influence of fashion should not be forgotten, though. In England, circumcision was socially approved of at the end of the nineteenth century and nearly all male babies were operated on until after the Second World War. In the United States the practice goes in and out of fashion.

Gay men are divided between those who prefer their meat "cut" and those who prefer it "uncut." A man who is uncircumcised has to take greater care over cleanliness, making sure that the skin beneath the foreskin is scrupulously washed. If it is not, a natural secretion called smegma will collect beneath the foreskin, causing a foul odor, much discomfort, and possible infection.

EARLY SEXUALITY

We are sexual beings from the beginning. In the West this obvious truth is often negated, because many people are frightened or feel threatened by sex.

To an infant, the sensory world is part of exploring, knowing, and understanding. All sorts of experiences are sensual for the baby or infant—from defecating and passing urine to putting things into his mouth to see whether they are hot, soft, nasty or pleasant tasting. Often there are negative experiences which go with the sensation of pleasure—wetting the bed or examining another infant's genitalia may bring a punishment of smacks on the bare bottom, which in turn can give another sensual sensation.

The majority of us undergo such experiences and forget them as we grow up, yet they can leave an indelible mark on the minds of some people. If explorations of adult sexuality prove disappointing, they may cling to their early memories and want to re-enact them.

Many of us find the greatest erotic stimulation is to be hugged and kissed by our lover. Affection, in fact, is the erotic turn-on. Were we kissed and hugged by our parents? Did we have our first erections as infants surrounded by this fleshly warmth? A great many children do not have loving and affectionate parents, and it is no wonder that these people, once adult, are sometimes turned on by other scenarios. The gay world has always been indulgent of fantasy and game playing. (See Toys, page 129)

Most gay men realize in childhood or infancy that they are attracted to the same sex. This strange sensation is often difficult to identify because it occurs gradually. Most people ignore it and suppress the knowledge until late adolescence when it becomes so strong that they have to acknowledge their feelings.

All children should be reared in an environment that teaches respect for the individual, whatever his sexual nature might be, allowing him to blossom without shame and embarrassment.

MASTURBATION

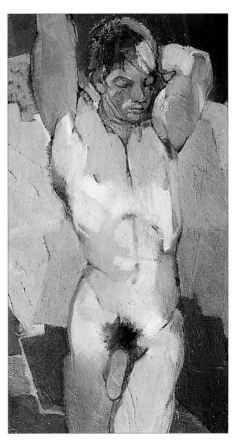

Until very recently this solitary sexual activity was frowned upon as being detrimental to health. In the eighteenth and nineteenth centuries, for example, it was thought to weaken and enfeeble the mind, eventually causing insanity. In 1878, Dr. N. Emmons Paine, a physician at the New York State Homeopathic Insane Asylum, published an essay which advised that masturbators be confined by a garment like a straitjacket, in which the genitalia were encased in a tin restraint. These views were not thought eccentric, but were accepted as part of a system of wise precaution. The doctor went on to suggest that, if these constraints did not bring about an improvement, the only hope was for the law to allow operations for castration without the permission of the patients' relatives. Such a law never came to pass, thankfully.

P.M., a nude by Cornelius McCarthy. Almost a modern St. Sebastian, the self-regard of the subject becomes a homoerotic communion of sacred and profane.

85

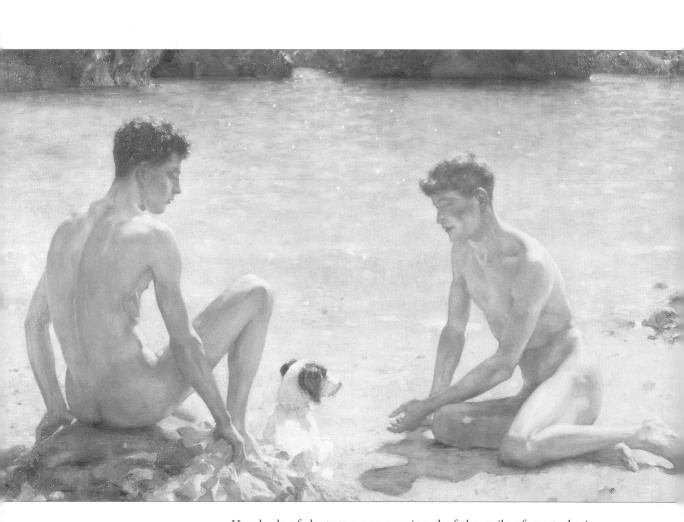

Comrades, by Henry Scott Tuke (1858-1929). Tuke and other painters of his time could paint naked lads without incurring suspicion, for even the discussion of homosexuality was suppressed.

Hundreds of doctors were convinced of the evils of masturbation and yet agreed that nearly all boys practised it. Unfortunately, illogic prevented them from asking why the asylums were not full of idiot masturbators. They agreed that masturbators were more likely to desire their own sex. So why did the majority of men grow up to become husbands and fathers, one might ask.

Why did people become so hysterical about masturbation, and see it as threatening the very fabric of their civilization? It is interesting to note that the horror of masturbation came into being with the birth of the homophobic state. In the minds of these doctors masturbation was

86

allied with a tendency to homosexuality. Many went even further and thought that if you were a masturbator, then you were sure also to be a homosexual. This assumption, as we know now, is completely false, and underlying it was the fear of homosexuality itself (see Persecution, page 100). Masturbation hysteria existed in Western society for nearly three hundred years—its origin can be dated to the late seventeenth century—and has only recently faded away.

In reality, of course, a boy who masturbates without guilt as an enjoyable release of sexual tension, as one of his sensual pleasures in life, is bound to be healthier and more balanced as an individual than a boy who is terrified of touching his own genitals. In fact, masturbation is a good way of beginning to explore yourself. It is perfectly possible to masturbate long before puberty; engorgement of the penis will occur throughout infancy and it can be massaged until a dry orgasm occurs. If the foreskin is tight, then it should be massaged very gently back on the shaft with the help of a lubricant.

MUTUAL MASTURBATION

This is probably the most common form of love-making, certainly at the beginning of a relationship, when two people are getting to know each other. It also has the great advantage of being safe. There is a natural and compelling curiosity to discover each other's genitalia, and to examine and fondle these most private of parts in all their shapes and moods can be enthralling, particularly when they so often reflect what is happening to our own body. Also, this very act of gently caressing your lover's genitalia reminds us of our first discovery of our own sexuality.

Mutual masturbation starts very gently. You may be naked or partly clothed, and lying side by side. In fondling the penis you will discover what your partner likes and which parts of the shaft and knob are the

Mutual masturbation is the best way of getting to know your partner's responses.

most sensitive. If you use a lubricant upon each other—an aromatic oil can be very pleasurable—you will find that by feather stroking the knob's rim with the very tips of your fingers will undoubtedly give the most delightful erotic sensations, and take you to the next stage.

Some people like their erect cocks to be rubbed throughout very gently, others like the rubbing to be quite quick and almost rough. Each person must learn this about his partner, and the best way is for each to show the other how he masturbates alone. Sometimes, however, left to ourselves, we tend to hurry things along, reaching orgasm too quickly. A lover may introduce us to a softer, slower method that is much more sensual. Feel free to experiment with each other, always considering, as you go into some new technique, what your partner is feeling and whether it suits him. Reaching orgasm at the same time can be learned. This is discussed in Simultaneous Orgasm (p.127).

FIRST LOVE

A boy's first love is often another male. He may be roughly the same age or an adult, very commonly a teacher. Often these loves are passionate but platonic, and do not become physical. Usually, when boys are young and inexperienced, they do not think of their emotions in sexual terms. These strong—and often painful—loves may remain platonic, nevertheless young boys may feel tingling excitement from being next to the beloved and taking delight in how he looks, the strength of his physique, or the beauty of his voice or his eyes.

Boys first explore each other's bodies very tentatively: this is the most natural thing in the world. After discovering the pleasant feelings they gain from the sensation of naked bodies together, they might even have fantasies about older men.

In the Judeo-Christian tradition, sexual love between adults and youths is prohibited. Because it is regarded as one of the greatest of all sexual crimes, punitive laws have been made against it. The ancient world, however, celebrated such love. For example, "Socratic love" love between a teacher and a boy was accepted as normal in Classical Greek society.

An adolescent with strong emotional feelings towards an older man must suppress these feelings or else create a situation in which the man is at risk of breaking the law. But suppression does not always happen, and affairs that result have to be kept secret from everyone. The two partners always have to be watchful and circumspect, which creates unhealthy pressure; the relationship will have to struggle to survive in the face of a judgmental society which holds that children are sexless and that the age of consent has to be in early manhood. (A few societies now exist in the world where the age of consent is equal between the sexes; in Greece, appropriately, it is fifteen; in Iceland fourteen; and in the Netherlands sixteen.)

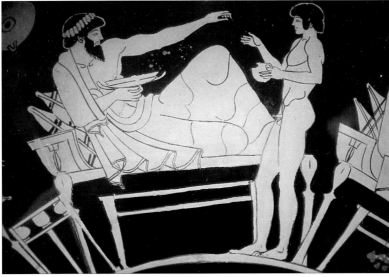

Man and youth at a symposium, fourth-fifth century B.C. Boys served wine and food and were often objects of interest and passion. Poems and letters were written in their honor and sexual activity might well occur afterwards.

The gay world believes, as did classical Greece, that such relationships are of enormous benefit. A youth so involved will learn much from his older lover, about moral values and being a responsible citizen. Often from such a relationship he will grow up to be a model husband and father.

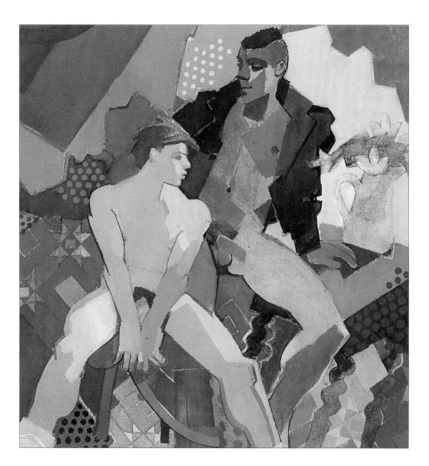

Johnny with White Boy, by
Cornelius McCarthy. This
painting catches beautifully
the mounting sexual tension
between the subjects.

FIRST SEXUAL PASSIONS

The first real love affair is unforgettable. Some people also spend a
lifetime lamenting the mistakes they made and grieving over the loss
of someone whose love they should have nurtured.

Because first-time lovers are young and inexperienced, they make
countless mistakes, which often seem silly and embarrassing later.
Thankfully, the fires of their passion blaze so fiercely that mistakes do
not matter. Sometimes, though, mistakes that accumulate cause major

quarrels which can end an affair that otherwise would have lasted.

The most common mistake in young love is to play psychological games, often without realizing it. The game usually starts with a real or imaginary hurt. The offended party might then pretend to fancy another man, or fantasize about some other love object. Then the first lover becomes truly hurt himself, and in return feigns another love interest, too. Thus a great web of pain and bewilderment is woven, each lover making the other feel insecure and unloved. It is the silliest game because both sides lose.

One part of the psychological game is called "the flounce," when at the end or in the midst of a quarrel one of the partners will flounce off and stay away. This is nothing but the spoiled child syndrome, where the child in a temper slams the door and refuses to speak. Such behavior in an adult generally passes in a few hours, but it can go on for days, weeks or months. Do not allow it to: insist on seeing your lover. Hug him and tell him how funny his behavior is. If you can show your love and make him laugh, he will return.

If we are lucky, we will refuse to be taken in by such games and keep from playing them ourselves. Regardless, the solution is always to tell the truth. If you are hurt by your lover's behavior, tell him at once. Do not allow it to poison you. Talk over every difference you have, explain why you feel hurt, and try not to keep things back out of pride or embarrassment. Only by revealing the whole truth to each other will you save your relationship. There is no reason why first love should not also be last love.

BISEXUALITY

Everyone has the potential to be bisexual. As human beings we respond to genuine warmth and affection from others; gender is secondary to the appeal and satisfaction of human touch. Our sexuality is very fluid, much of its energy lying within the subconscious. Society tends to restrict sexuality and put pressure on its members to conform to strict categories. It conditions people to believe that they must be heterosexual to achieve success and maintain the natural order of society. But, as we know, many children are certain they are attracted only to others of the same sex.

Many other children are aware that they are attracted to both sexes, but are taught by society that the only right and proper attraction is to the opposite sex. People are also born, or reared, to be natural rebels. To rebel in matters of sex is to strike at society's Achilles heel; therefore, a rebellious child will often be gay or bisexual or simply promiscuous. Society's hatred of "unorthodox" sex and its need to make laws against it indicates its vulnerability to sexual revolt.

We tend to believe that our sexual nature is somehow fixed, that whether gay or straight it will remain the same throughout our lives. But many people choose to be straight because it is so much easier socially. They suppress their gay desires, usually with little success, and attempt to live the lives of model citizens. Similarly, many gay people also suppress their heterosexuality because it does not fit into their image of themselves, or because they cannot fit heterosexual relationships into a gay life. The ancient world, where men had wives and boyfriends at the same time, was less complicated than today's society.

Some bisexual men and women do not find society as complicated as others. There are men who can happily go to bed one night with a woman and the following night with a man and find the experiences equally erotic. The erotic intensity of both exploits may even be heightened by the fact that one follows so soon after the other.

Bisexuals have a bad name because the gay world does not accept their behavior as genuine: it sees them as renegade gays. Straight society agrees with the gay world in this matter, and both automatically label men who are discovered to have had a gay experience as "gay," even though they might have wives and girlfriends. The happy bisexual simply does not fit in. Perhaps both societies feel threatened by people who can move so easily from one gender to the other; but there is surely nothing threatening about this. Having the potential of the whole world to choose a partner from, instead of just half of it, must be a happy state of affairs.

COMING TO TERMS

Our first love or sexual experience, having found our gay nature and being able to express it for the first time, brings great excitement. There is the triumphant, inebriating feeling of finding ourselves after so many years in confusion and darkness. We ally ourselves with all the great gays of history: with Plato and Plutarch, Michelangelo and Leonardo, Shakespeare and Marlowe, Byron, Tchaikovsky, and a host of others. We feel we are part of this great creative tradition, forgetting that half of these men were made miserably unhappy and anguished over their nature, mainly because of social persecution. (Plato and Plutarch were the exceptions because they lived in times when homosexuality was the norm. Shakespeare was bisexual, a condition which Elizabethan society found perfectly acceptable. Marlowe, too, was perfectly extrovert in his desires, as was the Italian painter Giovanni Bazzi (1477-1549), who signed his paintings "Il Sodoma.")

Negative thoughts come later, as we are forced to contemplate what we are. Finding our sexual nature is a great discovery, but there may be facets of it that we don't like and which we may suppress. But none of us should feel that our sexual nature is absolute and that we are stuck with it for the rest of our lives. Follow your instinct in this matter and explore further if you feel you need to. That exploration may well be toward other aspects of gay love, or it might be away from them, or it might combine them.

Many gays feel a loss because they might never father children. Increasingly now there are various arrangements that gay men and women make in order to have children and share their parenting. This could be explored by gay organizations, which should provide lists of gays who would like to conceive, raise and foster children.

The realization that one is gay can be so overwhelming that for

Opposite: Young Man against a Rose Tree, by Nicholas Hilliard (1547-1619). The Elizabethans accepted bisexuality without comment or censure, and the decorative and cultivated male flourished in the tradition of the *Kama Sutra.*

93

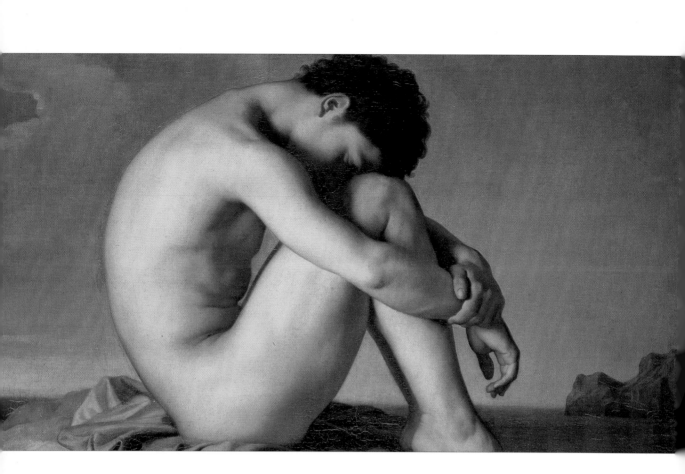

Naked Young Man by the Sea, by Hippolyte Flandrin (1809-64). This painting has become a gay icon; it was painted at the height of the Romantic period, and harks back to the male perfection of classical Greece.

years one is not aware of all the social factors which label one as a sexual minority and a threat to civilized values. Many feel sickened by the hypocrisy of their parents' values. Many show their disgust in some vivid way, perhaps by flaunting their difference in their clothes, make-up and hairstyles, in the music they play and the people they date. In the eyes of many parents, to "choose" homosexuality is to choose a sterile way of life. They see it as tantamount to saying that we do not want their familial line to continue. Though they may well have other sons and daughters, this perceived protest by one child strikes at their very existence. This is why "coming out" to parents can be so traumatic for everyone concerned.

COMING OUT

Once people are aware of being gay, they should "come out." This is hard, because they will be coming out to a homophobic society, saying, "I am one of those you spurn, hate and distrust. I am one of those men who you think deserve to be despised."

Remember, though, that our strength lies in straight men's fear. Deep within, they harbor the knowledge that they are capable of desiring the same carnal delights as we do. Any straight man placed for weeks in an all-male community will go with other men for sexual release and pleasure. They know we know this, which explains much of the tension between straight and gay men.

However difficult, coming out must be done. Do it with quiet dignity and modesty, and do not make a big deal about it. Though coming out to one's parents can be very difficult, depending on your parents' expectations of you, there are parents who, although surprised by your revelation, will cope well and will offer undemanding love and support. Alas, in our society such souls are rare.

Unfortunately, parents who have very fixed ideas and unrealistic expectations about what their children ought to be will always have problems with their children. It is far better for parents to want their children to fulfill themselves, however disappointing that fulfillment might be to the particular hopes of the parent. Truly loving parents will not mind in the least what their child is as long as he or she is fulfilled and happy. Coming out exposes the reality of the parent-child relationship: whether the parent actually loves him in an unselfish way, or whether the parent will only love him if he can be manipulated as the parent's puppet.

The mother and the father will probably react differently to the news. Both may worry

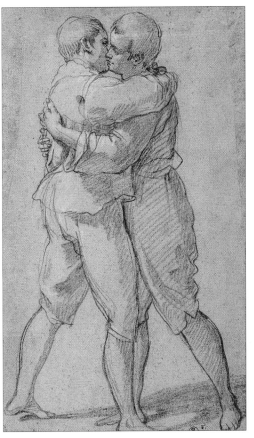

Two Young Men Embracing, by Bartolomeo Cesi (1556-1629). This late Renaissance drawing shows emotion being unashamedly expressed in public.

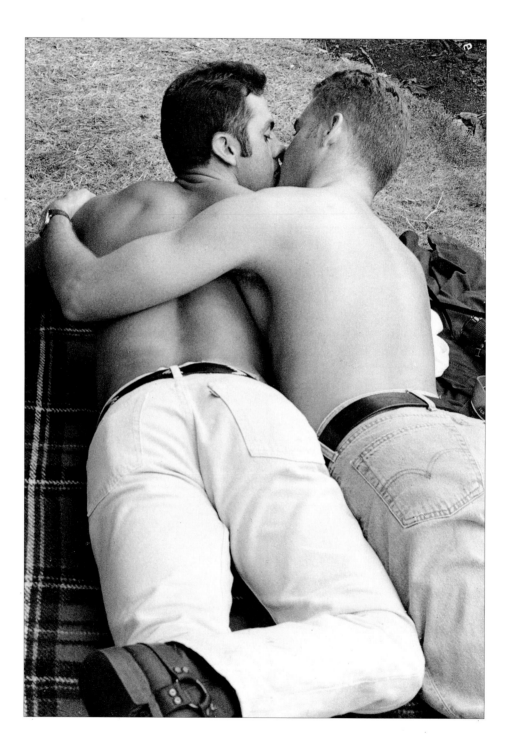

about the social shame, the lack of grandchildren, and AIDS. They may blame themselves for some lack of parental sustenance they should have given. Your job is to comfort and console on that point, and to alleviate any guilt they might have. Put your news in a broader context: give them some history of sexuality in other cultures, mention the findings of Alfred Kinsey (see p.114), or the fact that bisexuality was common in ancient Greece and Rome and that the human condition doesn't change that much in two thousand years.

Your mother may feel some warmth and kinship, and immediately start to worry about how your lovers treat you. She will give you dire warnings and tell you to take great care at all times. She has a point; be patient with her.

Your father may be more difficult, because to have a gay son is a blow to his social pride. How can he introduce you, he might think, to his colleagues as his son and heir, when they may know or suspect? On one level the thought of your sexual practices may make him uncomfortable, and evoke his own unspoken and unconscious sexual jealousy, because deep down he will not want any man but himself to enjoy you. He is unlikely to admit this to himself, however. So your confession may open a Pandora's Box for him. He may lose his temper and let out a tirade of fury, or say little and sink into depression.

The best way of dealing with such a father is to leave him alone. He will refuse to accept either your affection or your reasoning. In some cases it is wise to talk over your father's reactions with your mother. Women are often more perceptive about the human heart than men, and throughout their lives have to put up with the fact that many men can-

Opposite: Men showing their love and close affection is one of the most refreshing aspects of gay pride.

Below: Gay Pride Festival.

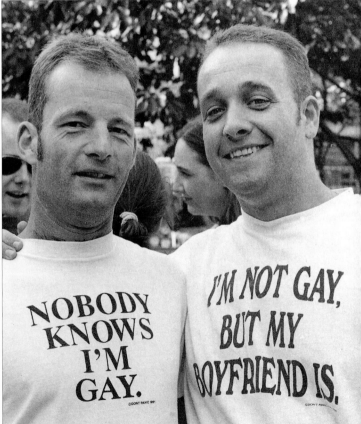

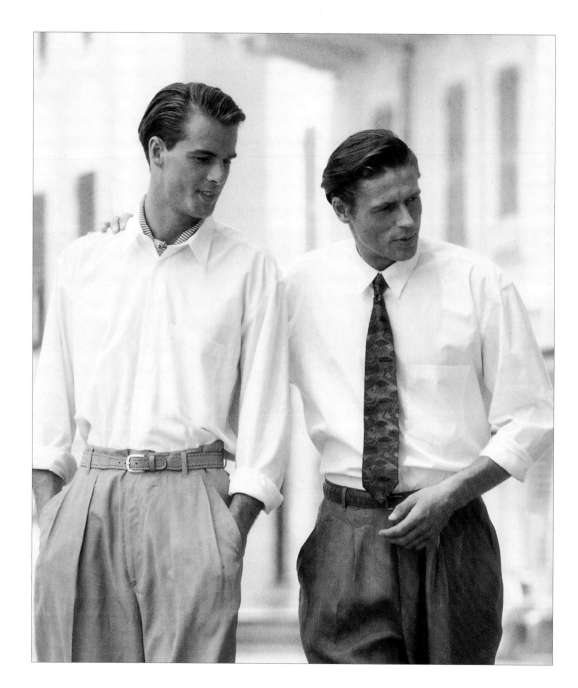

not talk about their emotions very easily. If you talk honestly about how you feel, it will delight your mother. She will probably be truly fascinated, and at the same time genuinely puzzled by her husband's behavior. If you can shed some light on the reasons why he is reacting so badly, your mother may well be able to transmit some of that information to him and enlighten him. A change in his attitude may be slow, so do not expect miracles overnight.

Some parents react so violently that they ban their sons from ever entering the house again. The hurt involved in such cruelty is immeasurable. A son of such parents should leave them to stew in their own remorse and hatred. A professional counselor can be of great benefit for the son, and the parents, if they can be induced to see one. There are also organizations which enable the parents of gays to meet and talk about the problems they perceive. These can be immensely helpful, but it can be a struggle to get the people who most need the help to attend the meetings.

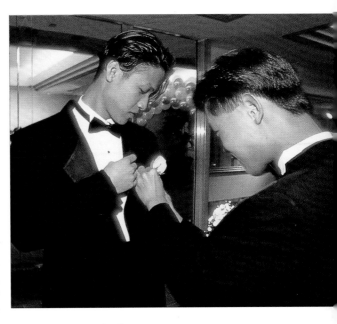

Coming out at work is usually simpler. When your colleagues talk about girls, just tell them that you prefer men. Once this fact is out, you will feel enormous relief. If they ask questions, tell them the whole truth. Such disclosures should be made to your peers rather than to your boss. Let the revelation permeate upwards.

After the news has sunk in, be watchful for any slights or derogatory jibes and stem them at once. Women in the workplace are often natural allies. If they protest against any sexist jokes along with you, with luck the straight men should be shamed into silence. But if such harassment continues, make a note of the remarks, the time and date and the situation in which they were made. When you have collected a small dossier of five or seven such occasions, make an official complaint to your superior or employer.

Above: First District sponsored Lesbian/Gay Senior Prom, Los Angeles, May 1994.

TAKING YOUR LOVER HOME

If after coming out you have a good and loving relationship with your parents, take your lover home to meet them. If you don't have a good relationship, do not even consider it. In this case, comment on the fact to your parents. Perhaps you can remark that your sisters' husbands are always well received. If you remain in touch with your parents, continually point out to them the inequality of social life and that you find their response unloving.

In the perfect home, you should be able to expect that your lover receives all the affection and understanding that a son-in-law is normally given. If they give you separate rooms when it would be possible to do otherwise, quietly insist on changing the arrangement. If they are worried about the attitude of grandma or other visiting relatives, tell them that you expected them to have been told. Grandparents are often, to everyone's surprise, quite amiable in their reactions to such news. They may well feel that at their stage in life it is too late to be shocked by such things and wonder what all the fuss is about. In such situations it helps to show affection towards your parents. A few jokes and a bit of sharp wit are also invaluable for improving the atmosphere.

PERSECUTION

Today vast numbers of people still persecute gays. They can be grouped into three areas: street thugs, the media, and politicians who enact discriminatory legislation.

An alarming percentage of the gay community claims to have been physically threatened or attacked, and murders of gay people have risen in the last few years. Extremely violent attacks routinely occur on the streets when gay men are set upon by gangs, sometimes beaten or stabbed and left to die.

With rising unemployment and increased poverty, many young men nurture great anger, frustration and resentment. They are only too happy to choose a convenient scapegoat on whom to vent it all. If these same young men have also failed to have a steady and fulfilling

Opposite: Gay love observes no barriers.

100

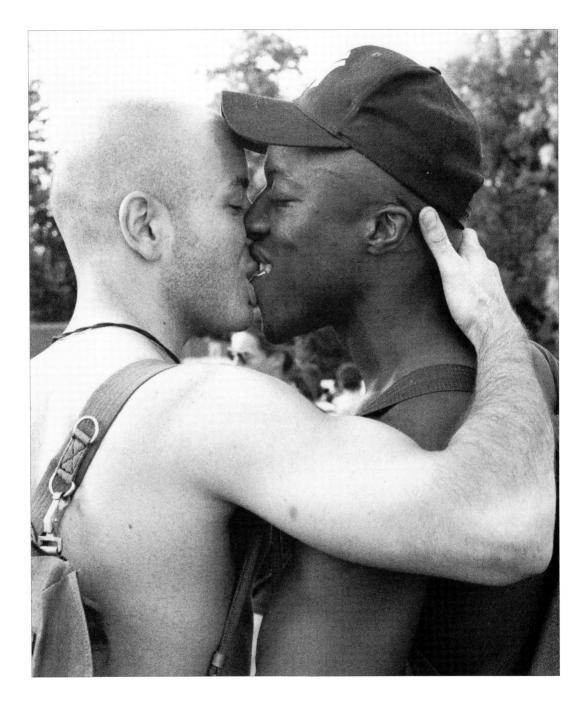

relationship with a girl, their sexuality is bound to be unhappy and muddled. Out of such confusion stems a hatred of the men who engage in unorthodox sex and seem happy about it, a feeling that they are perverts who are "getting away with it." Straight men may feel that these same perverts are somehow taking their strength away, and that only by attacking them will their own lives improve. Logic or reason has no place in their thinking. They may actually be suppressing their own homoeroticism. Anti-gay thugs would not exist without the bedrock of discrimination at the base of our society. Such thugs know that however evil and murderous their intentions and actions might be, in some respects society agrees with them.

Thugs bond often together with concepts of "buddy love," of being partners, like Butch Cassidy and the Sundance Kid, outlaws against society, who will do anything for each other. Such concepts hide and suppress the sexual element in friendships of this kind, and this very suppression fuels their hatred of gays. These "buddies" are killing what they fear in themselves, or what they may have already expressed.

Some murderers of gay men were once male prostitutes. When caught these men have based their defense on "homosexual panic," to which both juries and judges are often sympathetic. The charge of murder thus gets diluted to manslaughter, committed while the accused was defending himself against a sexual assault. At least one case has occurred in which a murderer killed again after serving only a few years for such a crime.

Gay people should stay away from badly lit cruising areas, and should not wait around outside gay bars, or cruise inside a bar or club. You can arm yourself with anti-rape devices such as high-pitched whistles, pepper sprays, etc. Used against four or five thugs these are very likely to be useless. Stay within your own gay group when crossing a dangerous area. Do not venture out to dangerous areas even in a couple, because two of you would still be an easy target for a group of thugs. Gay rights organizations should present a strong case for police monitoring of areas which are known danger spots for gays.

Newspapers and television programs often give space to anti-gay propaganda to profit from the anti-gay sentiments of a large section of

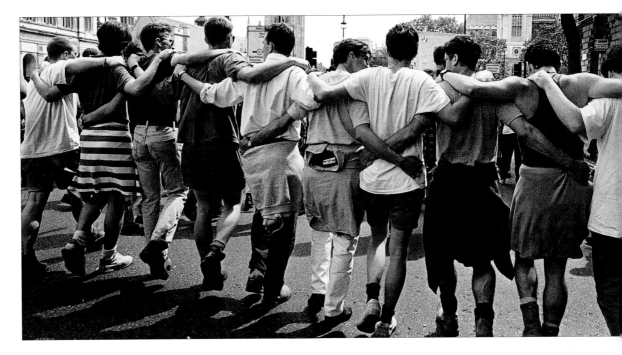

Entering Parliament Square. Gay Pride March, London, 1994.

the community. Such views are reinforced by much of society's legislation and by the religious beliefs of some clerics. They are presented with a gravity and high moral fervor which make them all the more pernicious. Discriminatory legislation sometimes goes back many hundreds of years and stays on the statute books unrepealed because legislators feel it would be a political liability to get rid of it.

The conservative elite has an irrational fear that homosexuality is sinful, and that uncontrolled sensuality will undermine "civilized values." When asked to define these values, they will answer in clichés such as "all decent-minded people are revolted by such behavior" or "in civilized countries such people should not be allowed to roam the streets" or "they need treatment" or "it isn't natural." And so it goes. We must examine these shibboleths and try to understand them, in order to defeat the homophobes.

We are living at a time of rapid social change. Many people cling to the values of the past, such as the idea of the family as an inviolate structure of permanent moral values. For them, homosexuality represents an attack on the very roots of the family. Such people often seem to think that the world would turn homosexual overnight but for their own restrictions against homosexual love.

103

THE BIBLE

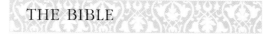

The homophobic arguments are often based upon crucial religious texts from the Old and New Testaments, conveniently forgetting the biblical text which says "the soul of Jonathan was knit with the soul of David, and Jonathan loved him as his own soul." (I Samuel 18.1) It forgets, too, that when both Saul and Jonathan are killed in battle, David laments and recalls that Jonathan's love had been "wonderful, passing the love of women." (II Samuel 1.26)

Some opponents of gays cite the Bible's prohibition of sodomy as evidence of the sinfulness of homosexuality. For instance:

"There shall be no sodomite [*kadesh*] of the sons of Israel." (Deuteronomy 23.18-19)

"And there were also sodomites [*kadesh*] in the land: and they did according to all the abominations of the nations which Yahweh drove out before the children of Israel."
(I Kings 14.24)

"And he broke down the house of the sodomites [*kedeshim*], that were in the house of the Lord, where the women wove coverings for the grove [*Asherah*, or sacred wooden post/phallus]."
(II Kings 23.7)

In order to understand the original meaning of these examples we have to strip away the distorting effect of numerous translations. We also must attempt to place the Hebrew nation in its historical context.

In the King James translation of the Bible the word "sodomite" does not have the meaning we give it today. Then "sodomy" was a term which covered sexual acts of any kind, between people of either gender, which were not vaginal penetration in the missionary position. So to James I, for example, "sodomites" would have meant any sexually uninhibited men and women. (That he himself was also a sodomite was irrelevant, for he was beyond reproach by virtue of the divine right of kings.)

When Jewish scholars translated the Bible into Greek, in the third

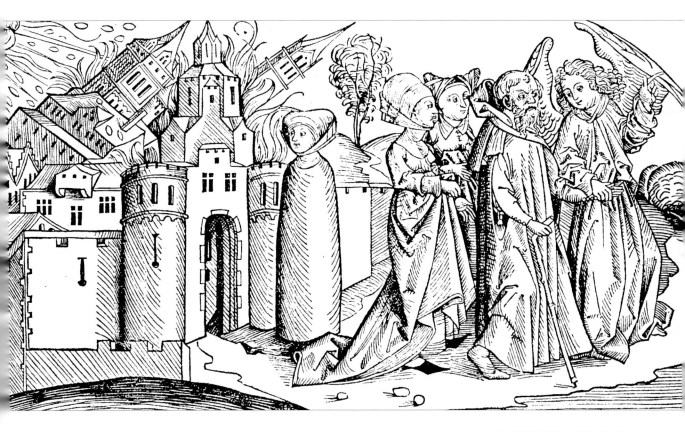

and second centuries B.C., they had great trouble in rendering the Hebrew word *kadosh* into Greek. (In Hebrew the word means "sacred" or "hallowed.") It proved such a problem that the translators chose six different Greek terms for the one Hebrew word, none of which would have suggested homosexuality to the theologians of the early Church who relied on the Greek translation. These passages given above were not used as condemnations of homosexuality until the mistranslation of the words into English in the early seventeenth century. By the end of that century the term "sodomite" had evolved to mean only one thing—a man who loves his own gender.

The destruction of Sodom and Gomorrah, showing Lot's wife turned into a pillar of salt. A woodcut from the Nuremberg Chronicle, 1493. There is evidence of a massive earthquake in the Dead Sea area in about 1900 B.C, and the legend of fire and brimstone could well have arisen from the escape of petroleum gases.

105

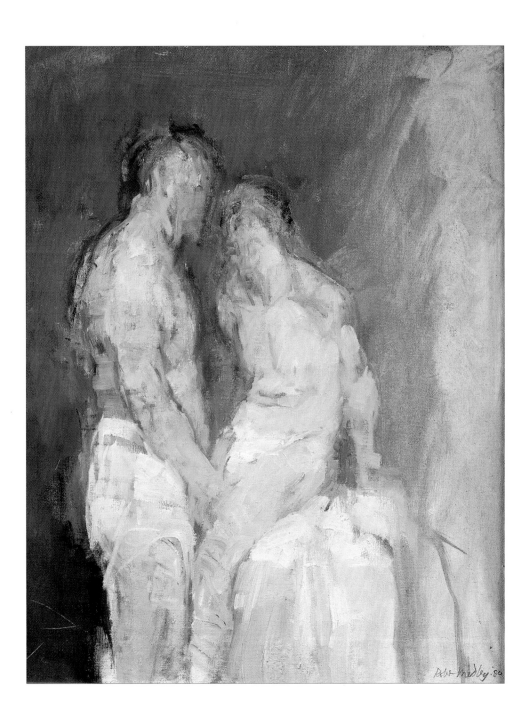

During the formation of the Hebrew nation, before and after the Babylonian exile, the people were surrounded by cultures which celebrated male temple prostitution. Hittite texts document transvestite eunuch priests. Babylonian and Assyrian texts refer to the priests who chanted, played music, wore masks and carried a spindle, a symbol of women's work. These priests, who were thought to have magical powers, had been castrated, and they submitted in the temple to rituals of anal penetration. In many parts of the Middle East religious traditions such as this continued until the advent of Islam.

Many of the Hebrew verses which exhort people to remove the sodomites are allied with instructions to destroy the idols. (The coverings which the women wove were for the phallus, which was decorated at different times of the year.) Israel, fighting a war against fertility ritual religions, set up an invisible God, a paternalistic figure who was warlike, aggressive and who laid down very precise laws of holy cleanliness. Many of these laws reveal a fear of the power of the phallus which still permeates societies today.

In the light of this history, the three verses quoted above are plainly admonitions against foreign male temple prostitution and false religious belief.

Another contentious text, "Thou shalt not lie with mankind, as with womankind: it is abomination." (Leviticus 18.22), also supports this interpretation. The Hebrew word *toevah*, translated here as "abomination," does not usually describe something deeply evil like murder or rape, but something which is ritually unclean, on a par with lying with a menstruating woman. The same Hebrew word is used when condemning temple prostitution and when calling the Gentiles unclean. When Leviticus was written, Judah was devastated as a consequence of the Babylonian exile (c. 500 B.C.): its cities were in ruins, the ruling classes had been deported, there were no kings and no leaders. But there were priests. The Holiness Code (Leviticus 17-26) is highly influenced by Zoroastrian purity laws, and so gives a structure for religious authority based upon sacrifices, purity and pollution. It says that if people will obey these rules, Yahweh will return to lead his people again. All the disasters, the defeat and the exile are explained by the guilt and sin of the people.

Opposite: Saul and David, by Robert Medley (1905-94). An interesting interpretation of the biblical story which depicts Saul's fascination for the young David as being one of physical enchantment.

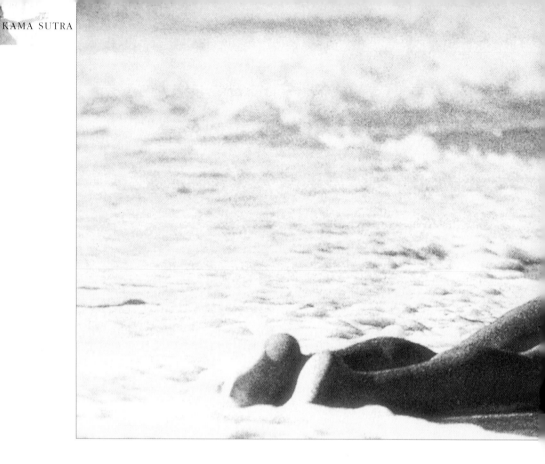

The Book of Genesis, which contains the story of Sodom and Gomorrah, is a compilation of various writers from different times. Some of it was written as early as 900 B.C., other parts in the seventh and fifth centuries. A thousand to fifteen hundred years separate the event and the story written about it. Furthermore, the incident on which the homophobic interpretation is based occurs after God has stated his intent to destroy the cities and all the people in them.

Two Angels arrive at the gate of Sodom. Lot recognizes them and invites them to dinner. The men of Sodom surround Lot's house and ask him to bring out the Angels so that they may "know them" carnally. The Hebrew verb for "to know" is very rarely used in a sexual sense; in only ten out of 943 instances in the Bible does it refer to carnal knowledge. Lot offers his daughters instead, but the men reject them and insist that the Angels be brought out to them. The Angels strike the men blind and inform Lot that the city will be destroyed in the morning. Lot and his family flee the city, and the story ends with Lot's daughters sleeping with him in order to conceive. Incest between father and daughter does not incur God's

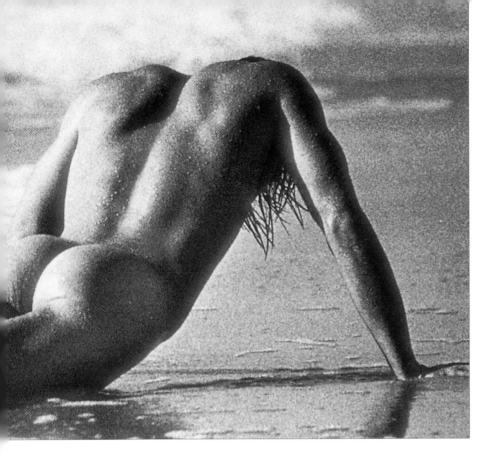

wrath, it seems. Yet homophobes cite this story as a divine law against homosexuality.

The early Church fathers did not interpret it this way. Origen and St. Ambrose both thought it concerned hospitality. As late as the fourteenth century, William Langland, the author of *Piers Plowman*, thought that the cities were destroyed because of sloth and over-indulgence.

In the New Testament homophobia bases its arguments upon several texts from St. Paul. Note that in the Gospels Jesus himself never makes any comments or judgments upon same-sex loving. In fact, throughout history various men—including James I, the French writer Diderot, and Leonardo da Vinci—have cited the love that Jesus had for his favorite disciple, John, as an example of their own love for some young man.

To understand the meaning of the Pauline texts one has to understand the historical context. Early Christians had to fight a plethora of different religious sects, many of them also disciples of Jesus. Many of these new Gnostic sects celebrated homosexuality as

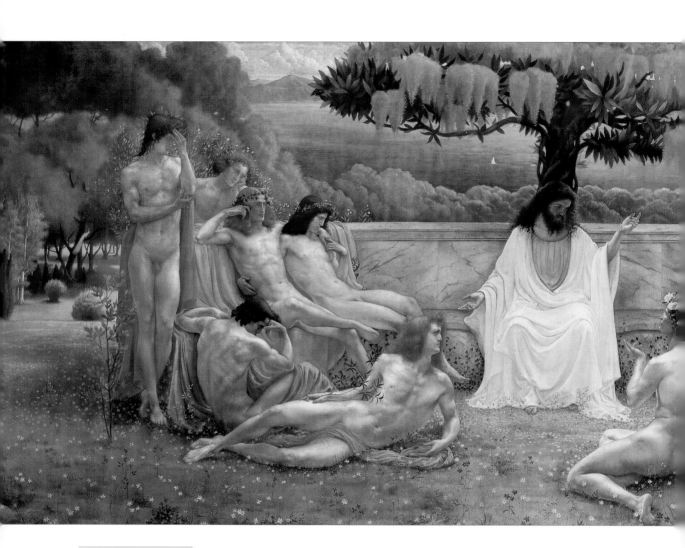

The School of Plato, by Jean Delville (1867-1953). An intensely homoerotic vision of the Platonic Academy. Notice Plato's portrayal as a Christ-like figure—connecting the early Church with the pagan world.

a means of becoming closer to God, in ways very similar to the Tantric Hinduism touched upon in the Kama Sutra.

Paul was a pious orthodox Jew up to his conversion on the road to Damascus, and his version of the teachings of Jesus incorporated Hebrew teachings. His views on women, for example, are misogynistic; he declared that they should always submit to their husbands and be silent. To Paul, women were the tribe of Eve, who had brought about the fall of man. He believed sex should be kept

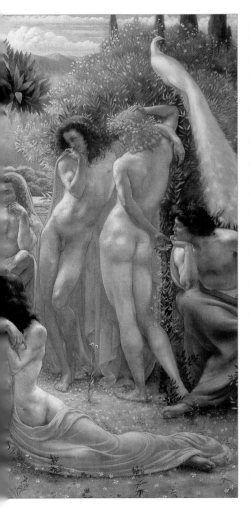

strictly within marriage.

In the time of Paul the Romans were the dominant culture and their ideas prevailed. They celebrated and extolled bisexuality. The eastern Mediterranean was dominated by Greek culture, with its emphasis on the beauty of youth. Timothy (I.1.9-10) details those in need of God's moral laws, including "them that defile themselves with mankind." The first chapter of Romans contains a tirade against men who burn with lust for one another, but this is specifically against pagans, who as we have seen celebrated homosexuality as part of their life and faith.

Down through the ages the Church has based its objections to homosexuality upon these texts, which did not always mean what is usually taught. The more fundamentalist the religion the greater its strictures against all forms of sexual expression outside marriage. This can be seen in both Judeo-Christian and Islamic religions.

After the death of Mohammed and as the Arab Empire grew, Islamic scholars created a detailed system of behavior called the *Hadith* ("the tradition"). There are now over 600,000 of these sayings which, not surprisingly, often conflict. The *Hadith* regarded all forms of sexual intercourse outside marriage, including homosexuality, as sins. Yet Arab society, before Mohammed and ever since, has been extremely relaxed about all kinds of sexual pleasures. Many Arabic poems and verses celebrate the love of boys. Throughout history when Christians visited Arab countries they wrote of the variety of sexual offerings.

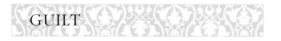

GUILT

Our lives can sometimes be devastated by feelings of guilt about being gay. Society creates guilt. If the individual is to succeed in releasing himself from his negative feelings, he must recognize that the guilt is not his fault. He has been made to feel bad because society needs a scapegoat. By making gay people feel bad and guilty, straights are attempting to eradicate the problem—that is, gays. In that they are preventing gay people feeling happy, they are certainly succeeding. The would-be gay son is made to feel bad by his parents' feelings and emotions. They embody society's anti-gay attitudes and pass them down to their children.

Some gay people feel guilty because their homosexuality causes their parents to be unhappy. This is the parents' problem; they are responsible for their reaction.

Guilt can become an underlying factor in other problems, such as impotence (see p. 132). If no reasoning from lovers or friends can help assuage it, advice from a professional may be needed.

NATURE OR NURTURE?

Are people born gay or does their early environment influence them? The debate is very old indeed. Recent research has attempted to discover a "gay" gene based on evidence of autopsies on the brains of homosexuals who have died of AIDS. All that was discovered was that a region on the X chromosome seems to influence variations in sexual orientation in men but not in women. Though this research is in its infancy and nothing has been proven, it seems to have opened up dangerous paths. If science has the ability to detect such differences within the embryo, then in the future it may be possible to wage a eugenic war against gays by screening embryos.

History itself disproves a biological difference between gays and straights. Are we to believe that all the males in the ancient world, in classical Greece and Rome, had this enlarged gland and that the majority of males now have not? Are we to believe that when an ado-

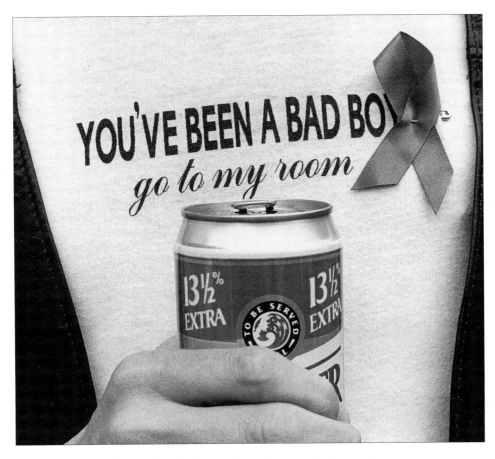

lescent has a gay love affair he has such a gland and when ten years later he is happily heterosexual the gland has gone?

The research into a "gay gene" seems to be an example of making the evidence fit the theory. The question to be asked is, why are scientists looking for a physical reason for homosexuality? Do these scientists want to be able to say that homosexuals are born with the equivalent of a club foot, for which they cannot be blamed, but which sets them apart from us? Thinking like this perpetuates the polarization of society into a superior group and an inferior group. We know which is which, but we should not accept such a patronizing attitude from straight society.

Gay people should not allow confusion to reign over the nature-versus-nurture debate. Let us declare what we know and not speculate for an entire community. People have different reactions to similar stimuli.

The sexologist Alfred Kinsey (1894-1956) pointed out that human beings are composed of male and female elements in a different ratio within us all. In his research he measured this ratio on a scale from zero, which was exclusively heterosexual, to six, which was exclusively homosexual. Most men and women clustered around the middle, at three. Given that we are a mixture of both masculine and feminine at birth, and given that all of us know masculine women and feminine men, why cannot the world accept bisexuality without qualms? Until recently, the world did accept it, and thought same-sex loving natural. No one worried about it.

Disparate types of people cohere to create what we call civilization, in which people work together for aims of common good. (Historically such groups have usually had a religious ethic to bind them together.) In order that a large number of people may coexist in relative harmony, laws are made to constrain our selfishness and enable a more thoughtful and caring society to emerge. These laws limit the freedom to commit murder and theft and punish transgression; other laws require us to share a proportion of the fruits of our labors for the common good. What society expects of its citizens changes all the time as various factors in human endeavor mold it.

As we mature we have to channel the rich complexity within us into some simpler form that will fit with society's norms. Most manage to do this out of fear; people are afraid that if they show their real selves they might be punished or made to feel deeply ashamed. Even children, because of environmental influences that they see with their own eyes, start to mold themselves into the kind of future citizen that society rewards.

If both nature and nurture mold the adult citizen, they certainly mold his or her sexuality. Although sexuality is partly a social construct, it flowers out of our earliest experiences. It is very difficult for each of us to name the exact influences because they start at birth. Generally, our sexual nature is apparent to us by late childhood, if not before. Unfortunately, as sex is still very much a taboo subject, such a revelation is rarely discussed and brought out into the open.

CAMPAIGNING

Secondary to the demands of love, no activity is more urgent than the campaign for equal rights. It is the very essence of the Indian concept *artha*—the relationship that links you with society and determines how you are judged by it.

Homosexual behavior is illegal in seventy-four out of the two hundred and two countries in the world. Fifty-three of these countries are predominantly Islamic, were formerly communist or were once part of the British Empire. The situation for homosexuals is worst in Africa and on the whole best in Europe.

In fifty-six countries gay movements exist and in eleven of these a

Homosexual marriage ceremony in Denmark, sealed with a kiss.

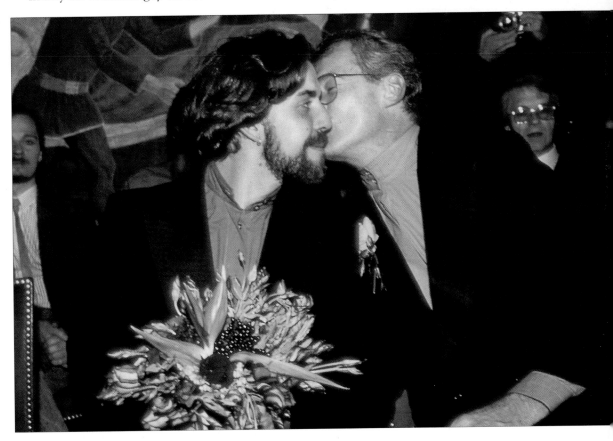

115

majority of the population is in favor of equal rights. In ninety-eight countries homosexual behavior is not illegal, although different ages of consent exist for gays and no laws prevent discrimination. In only a few countries (Denmark, France, Netherlands, Norway, and Sweden) does the law protect gay men; such protection also exists in some of the United States (California, Connecticut, New Jersey, New York, Massachusetts, Vermont, and Wisconsin), Canada and Australia.

In Islam generally one of the the worst possible sins imaginable is homosexuality. Punishment is whipping, stoning, and chopping off hands and feet of offenders. In Saudi Arabia punishment is the death penalty. Reports exist of individuals in China being given electric shock therapy.

In Europe and America the struggle for equal rights in society and in the eyes of the law still has a long way to go. No international human rights treaty explicitly distinguishes the rights and freedoms of gay people. Discrimination exists because the majority in most societies still consider gays to be sinful, unnatural, shameful, and dangerous to the family.

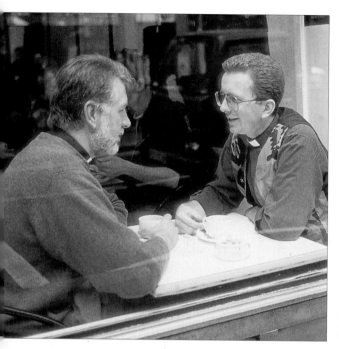

Anglican vicars in a gay bar. The Church of England is divided on the question of physical love.

Homosexual partners should have the same social rights as any heterosexual couple or man and wife. That is, if one partner dies they should have the right to all the property of the late partner and not be thrown out of the house by the family of the dead partner. They should have the pension rights of the late partner. Gays should have the right to privacy, their photographs, diaries and correspondence should be protected, and not, as now, perused by police to be used as evidence against them. Laws should ensure equal opportunities at work and in housing. The age of consent should be the same as for heterosexuals.

Gays have a duty to join organizations which fight homophobic legislation, and to use non-violent means to achieve equality with straight society.

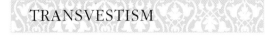

TRANSVESTISM

Transvestism is a person's desire to wear the clothes typical of the other gender. In women, it is not especially obvious because since the 1920s they have been wearing pants without society thinking it odd. Transvestism among men is more pronounced. They will often say how free they feel wearing a skirt or having silk next to their skin. Some men are very stylish, choosing their clothes with great taste, and are difficult to detect. Others are obviously men in feminine apparel, perhaps making a political point about the irrelevance of clothes and gender.

Transvestites need not be homosexual, and in fact quite a number are happily married with families. Wives who find such behavior diffi-

Camping it up in the desert. A scene from the film *Adventures of Priscilla, Queen of the Desert.*

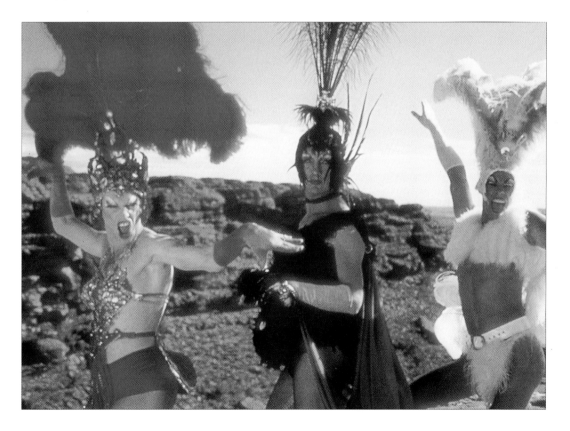

cult, however, are not to be blamed; they are only reflecting society's thinking of gender in absolute, rigid terms. The emphasis on masculine clothing is a matter of semiotics signifying gender. In the past masculine clothes were a mass of lace, silk and velvets, and often far more decorative than women's clothes. The men who wore them were no less masculine than their forebears or their descendants. The last great period of over-decorative masculine dress coincided with the Restoration court of Charles II in England and the court of Louis XIV in France. This was a time of sexual licentiousness when bisexuality was rife. It immediately preceded the birth of modern homophobia.

Once in Native American societies, a young boy or girl who wished to cross over to live the life of the opposite gender could do so without attracting adverse comment or ridicule. The child would dress according to the chosen gender and take up all of that gender's duties, including sexual ones at adolescence. He or she might live his entire life in this way, or change his or her mind at any time and switch back again. Native American culture respected the individual's decision and also revered the broadened perception such a change gave. Such an individual often took on the role of shaman and guru. The first colonists were often shocked at the practice, and called such people "berdaches," from the French *bardache* or the Italian *bardaccia*, meaning catamite.

Transvestism also occurs among gays. But where does one draw a line between the wish to dress as a female and transsexualism—the instinctual knowledge that one is encased in the body of the opposite gender? Going in drag, for fun, to a party is not the same as the desire to be dressed as a woman all the time. Gays naturally want the freedom to dress as they please at any time, without society making judgments on the suitability of a dress code.

How gay transvestites dress does not necessarily indicate what they do in bed. Some will only wear male clothes for work and be in drag the rest of the time. They may well have a "butch" husband and play the "female" partner in and out of bed. But other gay transvestites can vary their repertoire and take the active role. Clothes, in this case, do not make the man.

Opposite: Terence Stamp, looking good in *Priscilla*. Cross-dressing can be used as a social weapon to attack bigotry and prejudice.

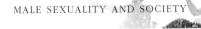

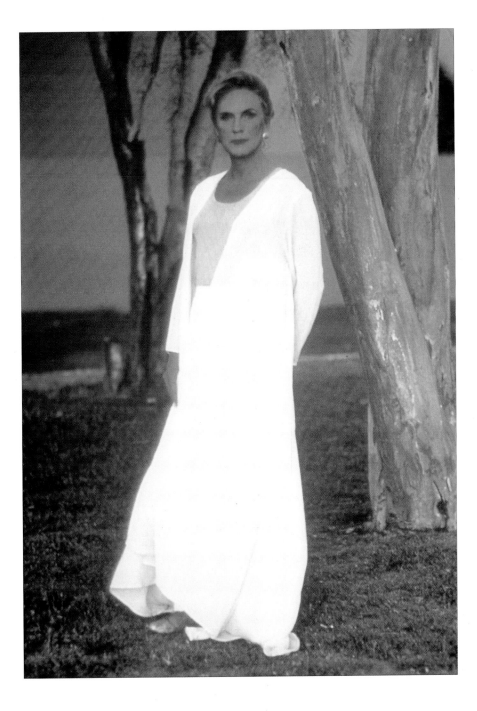

TRANSSEXUALS

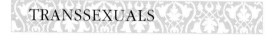

Transsexualism is when a man or woman has a powerful, instinctive belief that they are truly the opposite sex. It usually occurs when a child's sex is doubtful at birth and has to be determined by doctors through drugs and surgery (see below). Many such cases exist.

We have seen that some societies have allowed men and women to dress as they please. Cross-dressing occurs with much more frequency in societies where the genders are nearly equal. In societies where women are given little freedom, few men cross over to become female. To do so in such a society would be to choose a considerably lower quality of life. In Judeo-Christian and Islamic societies, where great emphasis is placed on gender distinctions, and clothes to reinforce those distinctions, transvestism and transsexualism are virtually unknown.

In the affluent West today, the social construct of womanhood is touched by the glamour of Hollywood. Advertisements present us with slim beauties, their well-defined curves draped in gorgeous clothes. These artificial and unreal women are the objects of straight male desire. Many gay men fall in love with such icons too, but they want to become like them. They may fantasize about straight men falling in love with them, but underlying their fantasy is a positive identification with their own gender. They are proud of their male genitalia, and comfortable within their own bodies.

Transsexual men are not comfortable at all. Many of them maintain that, although they want the hormones and the operation, they are not gay. Indeed, like transvestites, many of them have been married and fathered children before they discovered they really wanted to be women. After the operation, these men, now feeling they are women, will relate in love and sexuality only with men.

Have these men been so indoctrinated by society's fear of homosexuality that they have sublimated and rationalized their attraction to other men into a conviction that they must be women? Do they mistakenly believe that *only* women can be attracted to men? Their intense desire for surgery suggests a loathing of their genitalia. Yet cutting off the male genitals does not suddenly make a woman, as they discover. Though in time they may well have happy and fulfilled relationships, they choose a lonely, difficult path.

A transsexual will begin his sex change by explaining his feelings to a doctor, who will refer him to a special clinic. He will undergo psychological examination over two or three years. During this time he may start taking female hormones (which he has to keep up throughout his life). Then his beard is removed through electrolysis. The hormones cause his breasts to swell and redistribute the fat over his body, so that his figure becomes more curvaceous. He is then ready for surgery: the penis is split and turned inside out to become the vagina and a new opening is made to connect with the urethra. Once the flesh has grown and the body healed, it is possible for transsexuals to have fulfilling sexual encounters and to experience orgasm.

There is a medical condition found in newborn babies called Androgen Insensitivity Syndrome (A.I.S.) in which infant girls have male sex chromosomes, internal testes, a blocked vagina and no ovaries or uterus. Because the infants look like normal little girls, most parents will opt for them to keep that gender. Yet, they have to have female hormone replacement therapy from puberty throughout their lives and surgery to take away the testes and more surgery to make a proper vagina. At birth these infants could as easily have become little boys. There are also cases of infant boys whose penises are so minute that they have been mistaken for clitorises. Nature itself is not as clear about gender as society would like it to be.

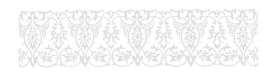

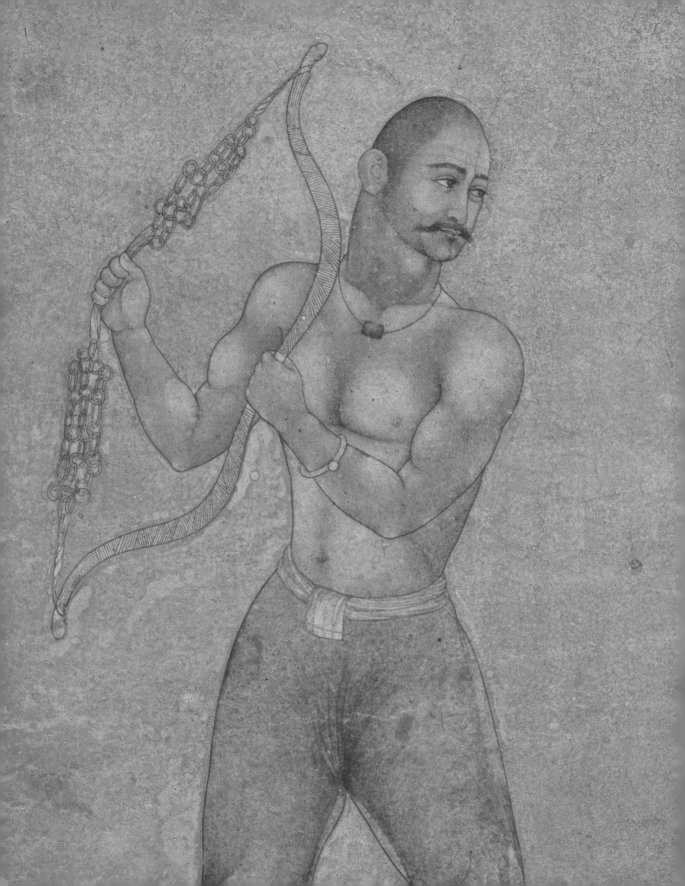

CHAPTER FOUR
SEXUAL GAMES AND RISKS

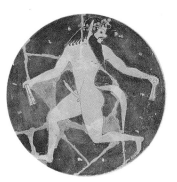

SHOWERING TOGETHER

Showering together is one of the most common sexual games. Soap foam is wonderfully slippery, and will allow orgasm between the thighs, if not anal penetration itself. Feeling each other's bodies beneath jets of hot water and soaping each other can be a lot of fun. Almost inevitably one partner will fill his mouth with hot water and go down on the other.

Sitting in the bath tub together also offers a sensual experience—though take care not to overflow the tub and cause a flood. One lover can sit on the other's prick and, buoyed by the water and gaining leverage on the end of the bath with his feet either side of his lover's head, can move his body up and down.

Opposite: Wrestler stretching a steel chain bow. This painting, dated 1700, presents a forceful image of Eastern masculinity.

Above: A Greek vase painting showing a dancing satyr, fifth century B.C.

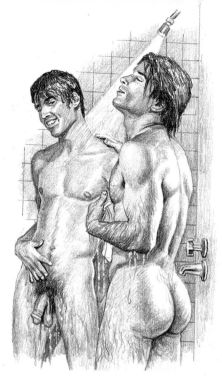

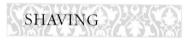

Living together brings more
intimate pleasures.

SHAVING

Wanting one's partner to be hairless, especially around the pubic area
and loins, is a common desire. All the hair around the genitals and on
the thighs close to and beneath the scrotum and up into the cleft of
the buns is shaved off. Sometimes this desire for hairlessness extends
to having all the chest and head hair removed as well.

A shaven adult body can be strikingly erotic. When it is also well
oiled, the combined look and sensation are amazing. Generally the
lover will want to keep the hairlessness in view during sex to remain
aroused, and positions will be chosen with this in mind.

One psychological explanation for shaving (if one is needed) is
that it has to do with our first sexual experience being pre-pubertal,
either with ourselves or with another. Through shaving we are simply
recalling the experience of an early childhood love.

Shaving is sometimes done as part of a short-term celebration of
love, perhaps for a weekend, and the hair is allowed to grow again.
Some lovers, though, will want their partner to remain hairless all the
time. If this is a demand that you are happy to comply with, you will
have to shave every few days to avoid the discomfort and scratchiness
that inevitably arises as the hair begins to grow back, especially on the
pubic area.

The act of shaving can be highly erotic for both partners. The presence of a razor (even a safety razor) near such a precious organ can

stimulate the lovers to greater heights. Take great care while shaving these tender parts and never forget that blood is an AIDS carrier. A sensible precaution is to begin by cutting away most of the hair with scissors and to use the razor sparingly to give a smooth finish.

If both partners shave off their hair the erotic effect is heightened still further, because both can enjoy the strange sensation of hairless oiled limbs and parts slithering over naked skin. The prick is, of course, hairless and smooth, so pressing it close into another's hairless body complements the overall experience particularly well.

PORNOGRAPHY

The difference between eroticism and pornography is not absolute because what is erotic to some people is pornographic to others. Gays would benefit from a definition of pornography to preserve their own notions of eroticism, but it is unlikely that gays would be any more successful at reaching a consensus than straight society. That said, there does seem to be a fundamental difference of opinion between gay and straight society over what constitutes pornography. Many straight people, for example, consider any depictions of erections as pornographic. What is so frightening, threatening, or obscene about an erect cock? The ancient world depicted erections all the time in its statuary, jewelry, and paintings, and gay men have regarded it as an object of beauty for centuries.

Gay society might be prepared to accept the following definition of pornography: any depiction of the domination of children for sexual pleasure, or of sexual violence, rape, or vicious humiliation done in earnest and not involving S & M playacting (see page 131). Depictions of sexual acts, of whatever kind, enjoyed by participants who have freely committed themselves would generally come under the label of erotic.

Such erotic material can be shown in magazines, videos, or live sex shows. They can be regarded as entertainment, and a way of adding extra pleasure to our sexual lives. Magazines and videos are often used as masturbatory aids.

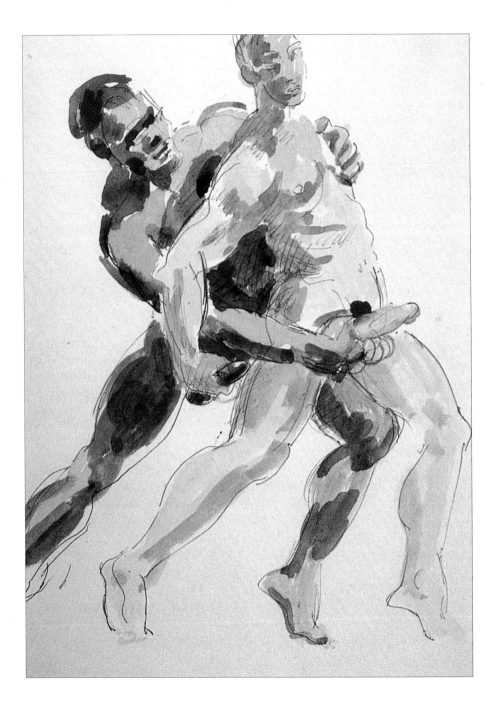

SIMULTANEOUS ORGASM

Also called "Twin Jets," this is hugely fulfilling and can occur almost by chance at first. With partners who are well attuned to each other, it can happen without them trying. If it doesn't happen, it is part of good sexual etiquette to attempt to contrive it, by one partner holding back until the other catches up. The penetrator holds the key to simultaneous orgasm. He can ensure his partner maximum pleasure by staying motionless inside him and delaying his orgasm for as long as possible. The position and the technique will, of course, determine how easy this is to do. Dialog is necessary to find out how near your partner is to coming, if you cannot trust your sensitivity to the signals given out by his sighs and groans. Co-operation and consideration are essential.

A selfish lover who fucks like a buck rabbit and does not care how his partner reaches orgasm is not a man most gays would want to sleep with twice. However, if this happens in a new relationship in which everything else seems fine, don't be afraid to talk about it. Such behavior could just be a sign of inexperience. All that's needed is some discreet advice and a wiser, guiding hand.

ORNAMENTATION

The tradition of wearing decorations which pierce the ears, nose, nipples and foreskin, or even the head of the prick itself, is as old as mankind. In some societies beaded sticks were threaded into a boy's penis and the skin allowed to grow around them as the boy grew up. The small protuberances added to the friction of intercourse to give the woman pleasurable pain.

Nowadays gold rings are worn in the ears, nose, forehead, the nipples and upon parts of the prick and scrotum. Rings placed in the nipples and upon the genitalia can heighten arousal for both partners. Pulling, tugging, biting, and nibbling them and the skin directly beneath can be immensely pleasurable.

Wonderfully intricate designs of savage and primitive beauty painted on the body are fun for a party or an orgy. The naked flesh of your

Opposite: Hercules and Diomede 2, by Duncan Grant. The sexual act is seen as a dance.

lover can be painted with scrolls, circles, snakes, birds, beasts, dots and lines, all in brilliant primary colors, so that he looks like a warrior from a primeval forest. When confronted by such a vision, one can savor how male desire and male love must have been in ancient times. Use paint which does not rub off easily, so it does not spoil interior furnishings. Theatrical make-up is the best.

Make-up is a means of enhancing the beauty of a naked man before a bout of love-making. The nails of the feet and hands can be painted, and the face itself can have a maquillage in the traditional manner. The face should not be excessively made up; you are aiming for a subtle effect simply to enhance the natural manliness that is inherent. The eyes can be dramatically outlined and a simple but very scant costume worn. Jewelry will look appealing if worn on the neck, over the chest, and around the waist. The genitalia can be decorated with beads, flowers, silk ribbons, fringes, tassels and jewels. The Roman emperor Commodus always had a naked boy covered in jewels beside his bed.

From here it is but a short step to costumes and wigs.

Lovingly decorating each other's body deepens the eroticism.

DRESSING UP

Gay fancy dress parties can be an excellent prelude to an orgy, especially if the theme is Roman, as togas can be thrown off easily. One of the most famous orgies in history was given by the Marquis de Sade in Marseilles. Ever the thoughtful host, he had the food spiked with Spanish Fly (see page 172). Legend has it that the lust was so great that four hundred and fifty people were fucking all night long and were never satiated. So far, no one has attempted to mark the anniversary of this party with a similar celebration.

Dressing up for just two can be almost as much fun. Any attractive costume will do. Wigs, if they are long and luxurious, can add immensely to the appeal. The best types of costume are invariably those with the most heady sexual relevance—the tight pants and bolero of a toreador; the hairy pants and horns of Pan himself; the short tunic of a Greek athlete.

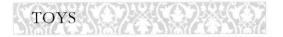

TOYS

If you use dildoes, make sure that they are scrupulously clean and well oiled before use, and that they are of an average size that will not harm you or your partner. Dildoes do have a practical use in relaxing the anal opening. A man who is nervous about being penetrated can experiment by himself with a dildo or a vibrator. Dildoes have been enjoyed for thousands of years. Many early civilizations (Sumerian, Chinese and Egyptian, for example) used dildoes. These were made from various materials: wood, pottery, bone and leather. In ancient Greece, a man named Miletus grew wealthy on the income he made from manufacturing and exporting them all over the known world.

Now, dildoes are generally made from rubber or plastic, both of which are easier to keep clean. Vibrators are battery-powered dildoes that shudder rhythmically when they are turned on. Some people find them very stimulating, while others are indifferent to them. Unfortunately, many vibrators are cheaply made, and can fall apart. Comparison-shop when buying one, and complain to the manufacturer if it is faulty.

Larger plastic or rubber dildoes can be used to beat the buttocks or other parts of the body, which many find highly arousing.

Cock-rings go around the prick and balls. When the penis is erect the cock-ring traps the blood so that the erection does not wane. Even after orgasm the erection can be maintained and the fun continued. Cock-rings must be tied quite tightly. The best kinds are adjustable, and generally made from leather or metal. The only real disadvantage of a plain, non-adjustable ring is that it is difficult to get off, because of the time it takes for the organ to lose the engorgement of blood. However, they look pleasant, they are not uncomfortable and they work efficiently. You can, of course, make your own cock-ring: just tie your prick at the base of the shaft with a ribbon or a cord, or even a thin leather belt.

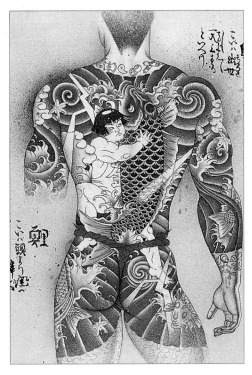

Kintaro 1/Carp Boy Tattoo 1.
A painting by the contemporary Japanese artist Sadao Hasegawa.

129

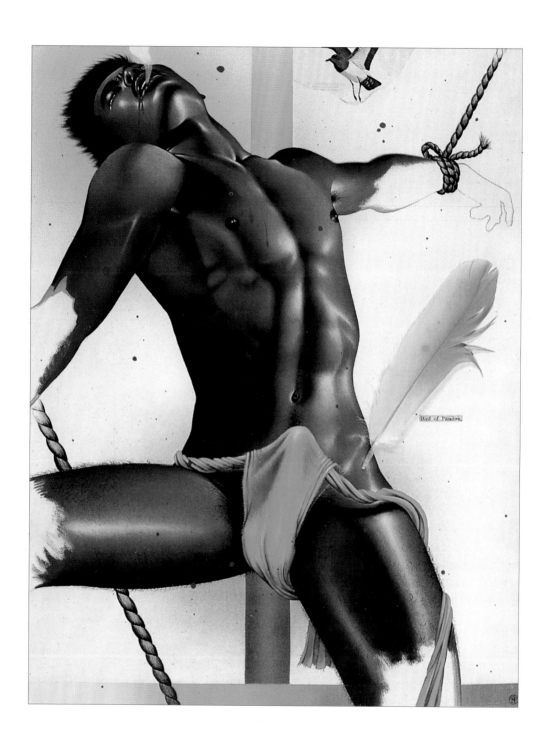

Bird of Paradise.

S & M

S & M stands for sadism and masochism. In the S & M scene, playing master and slave is the principal sexual activity. S & M is a diverse field which straight society also enjoys. Many of the activities are tame, though they may look terrifying. Black leather gear, buckles, straps, handcuffs, cock-rings and black leather head masks are common. Much of the sexual pleasure is gained in the playing of the roles rather than in the orgasmic climax.

Slaves often wear spiked dog collars and are held on leads. They may be handcuffed or tied to wall rings or bed-posts and immobilized. The masters humiliate, spit on, piss on, then whip and penetrate them. The pain a master causes his slave can be considerable, yet willingly the recipient will return for more.

In S & M, when real cruelty seems involved, it always arises out of the individual's own desire. The wish to be punished or to hurt someone may strike many people as bizarre, and should be treated responsibly. However, if men truly enjoy themselves in this way and are harming no one else in the process, they should be allowed the freedom to do so.

WATERSPORTS

This, or "golden showers," is the term used for pissing on your partner. This is a minority activity and usually confined to the S & M scene; a slave might be ordered to drink his master's urine or bathe his body in it. Another scenario in which watersports occur is when men are high (or otherwise incapable of erection or orgasm) and resort to drinking a lot, then pissing on each other.

Opposite: Impaled.
Hasegawa's charged painting of bondage echoes the European myth of the torture of Prometheus, the Greek hero who was punished for stealing fire by being chained to a rock, where his liver was eaten by an eagle.

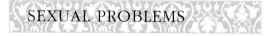

SEXUAL PROBLEMS

Impotence

Impotence, the inability to have an erection, can happen to all men, straight or gay, at any time of their lives. It can be caused by various factors, including sexual boredom. There is usually an easy cure: find some erotic material, or anything else that turns you on, and masturbate. If you achieve erection, there's nothing basically wrong. You just haven't found a partner who relaxes you and turns you on, or anxieties may be inhibiting you.

Impotence can also stem from tiredness or stress. Get some rest and take steps to reduce the stress in your life. The worst thing to do is to worry about the impotence itself; such anxiety will always increase it.

If your mind and emotions are engaged, but your cock still refuses to react positively, or only after a lot of manipulation, you may have deep-seated inhibitions about sex itself, or sex with that particular partner. Try to relax and talk it over with him or a close friend. Do not expect to get results immediately; you'll probably need a few weeks to work through it. Think about why you enjoy being gay, and why you're in love with that particular man. You will find the answers. Perhaps you love him but you don't trust him. Some people, for example, cannot fuck anyone they don't trust, and for them entering another person's body demands the ultimate trust.

If there is still no solution, do not despair. Go to your doctor. Do not let him tell you that your impotence is due merely to stress or tiredness. Only a thorough medical examination will reveal the physical reasons for impotence.

Premature Ejaculation

People who suffer from premature ejaculation miss out on all the fun. It can also be highly embarrassing if the orgasm occurs when fully clothed and a tell-tale stain is perceived. Luckily, sufferers can help themselves quite easily by becoming more aware of what is going on in their own bodies, monitoring their erection and then disciplining themselves to slow down.

Opposite: A narcissistic quality permeates much contemporary photography, showing the body beautiful alone and self-regarding, teasing the viewer with a glimpse of unobtainable fruits.

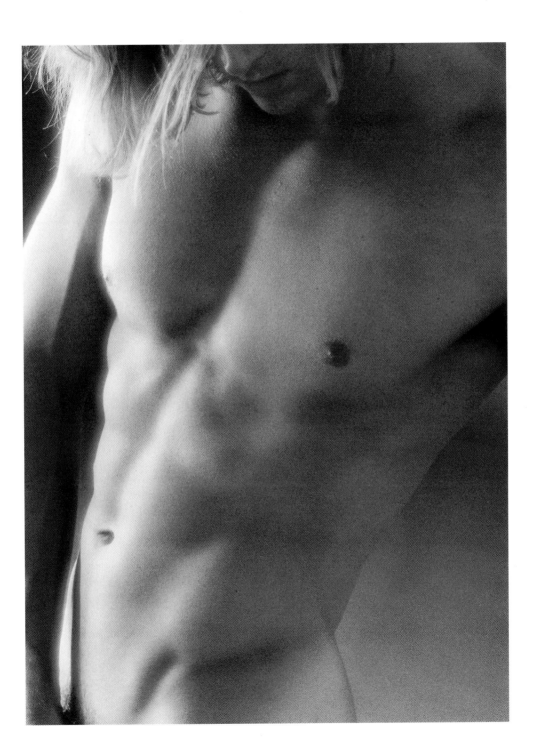

Being able to control the timing of the orgasm is the central part of the art of love. You can teach yourself to do this: masturbate until you feel you are about to come, wait a minute, and then gradually start again. Repeat this three or four times. You should be able to do the same when you are next with a lover. Premature ejaculation can also happen after a period of denial and chastity, and is not a major problem. If it happens, make love again and continue for as long as there is the need.

Rape

This is not just a heterosexual problem. Gay rape has for years been covered up and news of cases suppressed. It often occurs in all-male institutions, such as prison or the military, where it may be a one-on-one act or gang rape. The last few years have seen several cases of straight men being raped in public places at night. Some rapists add to their victims' ordeal by informing them after the act that they are HIV positive. If you are the victim of a rape, however ashamed or embarrassed you may feel about it, you must report the incident to the police. Male rape is now treated by the police with the seriousness it deserves and they will provide support services to help you. Whatever you think, you will need counseling. The forced intrusion into your body will leave you with deep feelings of uncleanliness, of being out of control and unable to cope with your own life. These feelings are absolutely natural, but you will need a professional to guide you through them and alleviate the shame and hurt.

Body Image

We are all dissatisfied with how we look. Even the most stunningly beautiful young man worries about flaws in his physique. Whatever failings we believe we have, your lover will probably never notice them, any more than you will notice or care about his. We are all imperfect in one way or the other, so stop worrying about it. Instead, concentrate on what you like about yourself.

If your anxieties about body image continue, confess what it is you cannot endure about yourself to your lover or your friends. Your revelation will probably astonish and amuse them at the same time. What you find unbearable about yourself they probably have not noticed or may genuinely like.

Feeling happy within your own skin is an important aspect of

Opposite: The man at ease and enjoying himself invites the viewer to partake of the experience.

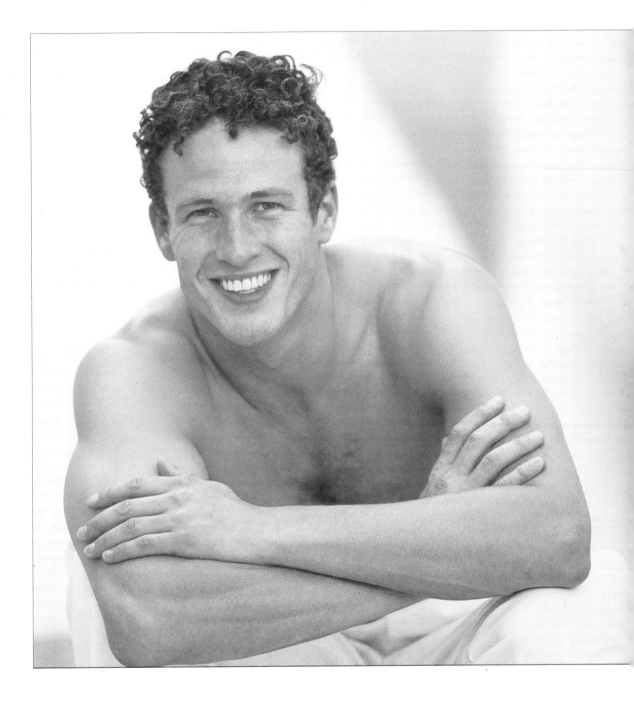

living. It affects your whole life, including the way you stand, move, sit and walk. If you are comfortable with your body, your attitude towards yourself will immediately be apparent to others. The impression that you live to the full within your body, exult in it, celebrate it and never abuse it, will invigorate and attract all who meet you. Being happy with your body is highly significant and will enhance your self-confidence and general sense of well-being.

Sexually Transmitted Diseases

Some infections have symptoms which appear on the genitals. If you see or feel anything unusual, examine it and refer to these pages or any other manual, then go to a doctor. If you are promiscuous, always practise safe sex (see p.65). Since the AIDS epidemic began, the rates of gonorrhea and other non-specific sexually transmitted diseases have declined very noticeably as gay people have heeded this advice.

AIDS

AIDS (see also page 66), or Acquired Immune Deficiency Syndrome, describes a collection of diseases which eventually lead to death. It is caused by a virus, or more specifically a retrovirus, known as HIV (Human Immunodeficiency Virus), which enters the body and attacks the human immune system. AIDS itself is not transmitted.

HIV, which eventually progresses to "full-blown" AIDS, is passed from person to person in certain body fluids: saliva, blood, semen, and vaginal/cervical secretions, and breast milk. Cases of HIV transmission usually occur as a result of unprotected penetrative sex (vaginal or anal) or sharing injection equipment. HIV-positive women can also pass the virus to a fetus through the blood.

Each different virus that attacks human beings lives and multiplies in a particular part or parts of the body (for example, the cold virus attacks the nose and throat, and the hepatitis virus attacks the liver). When these attacks occur, our immune system makes antibodies to fight the virus. But HIV attacks the immune system itself, gradually weakening it so that the body cannot fight off disease.

A person can continue to live with HIV for many years before their immune system is so damaged that they develop full-blown AIDS. Thinking positively, eating a diet with plenty of raw fruit and vegeta-

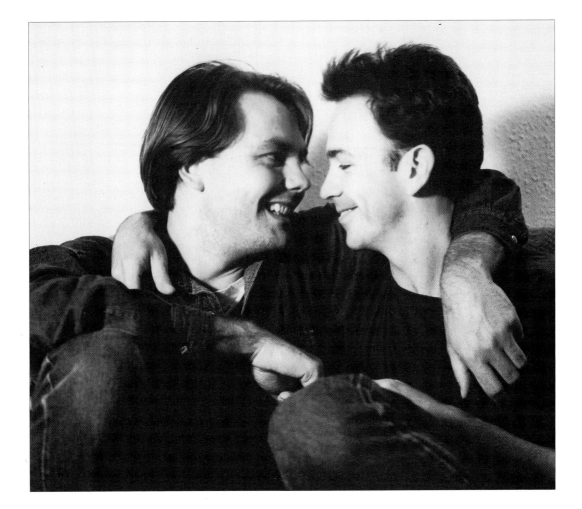

Gay couple. A picture of deep affection and happiness.

bles, whole grains and organic foods, and getting regular exercise, can be greatly beneficial.

There are no specific symptoms of AIDS, but the following may occur. Many patients have enlarged lymph nodes, or swollen glands, at several different places in the body. Some have unexplained and very severe diarrhea, with significant weight loss. There may be prolonged loss of appetite, profound and long-lasting fatigue, headaches, nausea and dizziness. Karposi's sarcoma, a form of cancer, appears as

137

a blue-violet or brownish spot on the skin. Lymphomas of the brain result in continuous or repeated bouts of blurred vision, headaches, mental disorientation, fits and personality changes. Pneumocystic Carinii has symptoms similar to other forms of pneumonia, such as a bad cough, chest pain and fever. Its main feature, however, is inexplicable and severe breathlessness.

If you are suffering from any of these symptoms, take immediate action. Go to a Sexually Transmitted Diseases (STD) clinic, where the doctors are specialized in the diagnosis and treatment of AIDS.

Safe sex involves avoiding forms of sex which can pass on infection and having sex in ways which cannot transmit the virus. Never have anal sex without a condom (unless see page 65), never share sex toys such as vibrators, and avoid all forms of sexual play and sadomasochism which draw blood. Play safe by going overboard on caressing, hugging and cuddling, massage, body kissing, mutual or group masturbation, thigh or buttock fucking. Always practise safe sex with strangers.

With a condom, always use a sterile, water-soluble lubricant such as KY-Jelly. When rolling on the condom, leave a spare centimetre or so at the tip to allow for the ejaculation and minimize the risk of bursting. Never use an oil-based lubricant such as Vaseline, or a body lotion, cold cream or baby oil because they may cause latex condoms to disintegrate.

If you are in any doubt at all about any past or present partners, it is sensible to have an HIV test and to repeat it annually. Unfortunately, the incubation period for HIV is unknown. It may be a few months, a few years, or even more. Thus regular HIV testing is the most sensible course to take.

Gonorrhea can show up in the penis or the rectum. An infection of the urethra, it will make itself felt between twenty-four hours and five days after you have been infected. Every time you urinate you will feel pain and your penis will exude a thick yellowish pus. Get treatment immediately from your doctor, who will put you on a course of antibiotic drugs. If you are infected in the rectum, the symptoms are constipation, rectal bleeding, and pus or blood in the stools.

Syphilis develops through several progressively worse phases. It first appears as a pain-free sore or canker on the head of the penis. The sore can also develop in the mouth or lips if you have performed fellatio on an infected person, or in the rectum, in which case you might not know it is there. It shows up ten days or even as much as three months after sexual contact. It is important to seek medical advice at this early stage. If left untreated, the sore will heal itself in about three weeks—but do not be deceived by its disappearance, for this is just the first stage of the disease.

Untreated, the disease goes on to its second stage, which takes about three to six weeks to develop. A rash will break out all over the body and you will want to vomit; you will have headaches and a high temperature. During this stage the disease is highly contagious. It is very important to get medical help and drugs. Left untreated, the symptoms will disappear after about a year, but again, do not be deceived.

The disease then lies dormant for anything up to twenty years before it moves into the third stage and fits one of three patterns: benign, giving you large ulcers; cardiovascular, which will end in heart failure; or paresis, where the infection attacks the central nervous system, leading to insanity or paralysis.

The minute a sore appears on the cock, seek medical attention.

Crabs are lice which live at the root of the hair follicle, nearly always in pubic hair. Because they itch horribly, you immediately know you have them. A close inspection of your pubes will reveal minute, crab-shaped lice. Several over-the-counter preparations can be bought to rid yourself of them. Simply douse the infected parts with the lotion. Continue the treatment once a day for three days to make sure you have also killed the eggs. Wash and disinfect everything you have used, such as bed linen, towels and underwear, to make sure you do not re-infect yourself.

Scabies are tiny parasites which you can't see with the naked eye. Again, the itching is unbearable. You will find it all over the body, wrists, fingers, ankles, crotch and between the arms, especially where

139

the skin is creased. Scabies are transmitted by contact with skin, towels and sheets. A doctor will give you a prescription for a lotion that will bring immediate relief.

Hepatitis is a viral infection of the liver and can be caught by kissing, or through the blood or semen. The symptoms are nausea, tiredness, aching and yellow skin. There is no cure for hepatitis, but you should be under a doctor's care nevertheless. You will have to give up all alcohol for at least six months for your liver to recover. Vaccines are available.

Herpes is a virus which produces highly infectious cold sores on the penis. They will go away after a week or so and might stay away for years before reappearing, but they are always with you. There is no known cure.

Venereal warts are a form of viral infection, transmitted through sex. The warts can develop in the rectum or just outside the anus or on the penis itself. They are unsightly but not painful. They can be removed in one brief, painless operation performed by a doctor, or treated with a prescribed lotion.

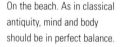

On the beach. As in classical antiquity, mind and body should be in perfect balance.

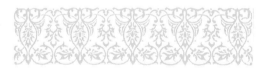

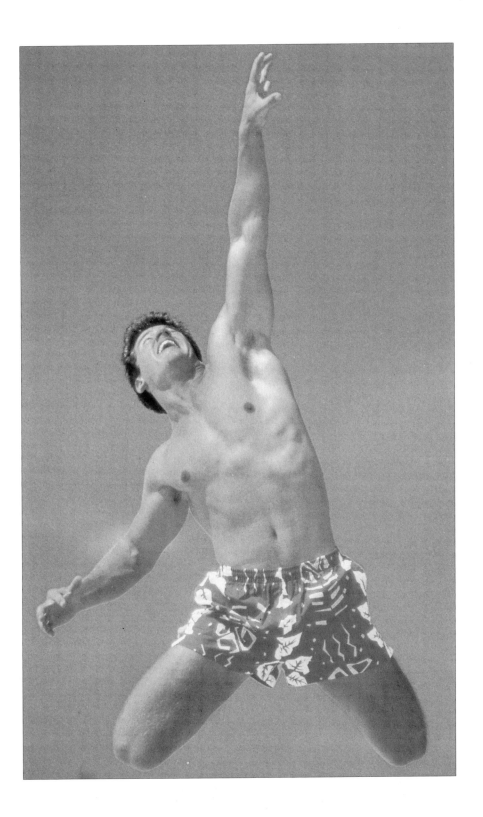

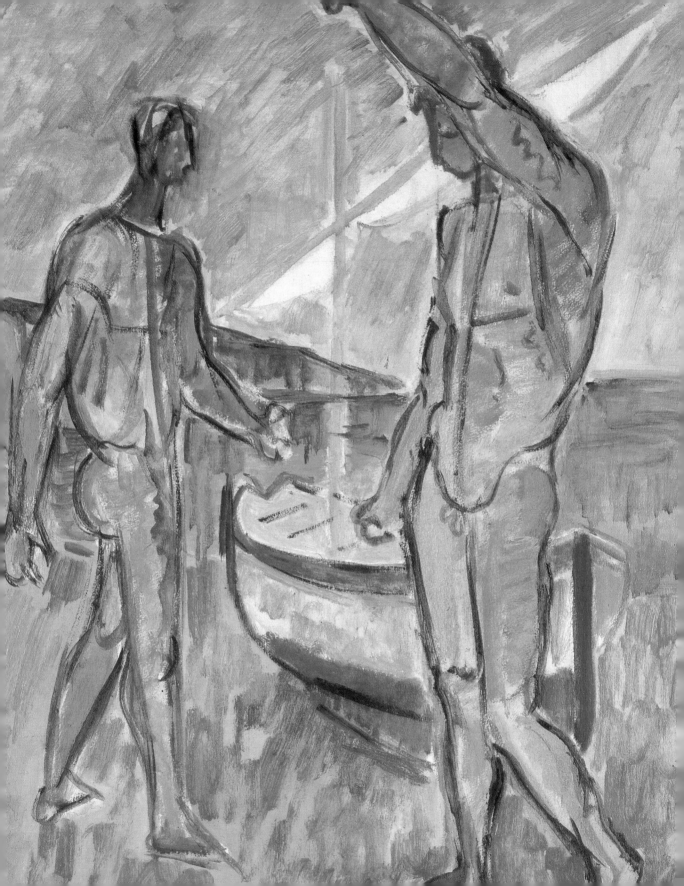

CHAPTER FIVE

ACQUIRING A PARTNER

If a man is true to himself and well educated in the arts and sciences and has many diversions, he will have earned the respect of his society. Such a man should have little difficulty finding himself a loving partner. But many a potential romance has been destroyed in the first few days by over-eagerness or a nervous disposition.

If the first sight and the first touch have occurred without either finding fault, be circumspect in the pace at which the romance is pursued. Encourage the pursued to talk about himself, especially his childhood and his family. Be a good listener. Absorb all the information, for it is a map of the journey he has already taken. Offer warm friendship towards all the friends he mentions in passing, express interest in his parents and family, and in his work and hobbies. Nothing else will be quite so seductive as your concern in these matters. However, your interest must be genuine; if it is merely a ploy towards seduction, you are deceiving yourself as well as him.

Be sure, too, that his interest in you, your childhood and family equals yours, for some men will soak up all such interest and never return one iota of it. Watch carefully in these first few days and weeks that the relationship is equal. See each other as often as you wish, make love tenderly, even sleep occasionally at each other's homes, but take it slowly. Try not to talk of the future; live for the moment.

Of course, many partnerships are unequal from the start. These are not likely to have a long life. Inequality of age, property, talent or wealth rests on one partner being dominant and the other becoming

Opposite: Two Fishermen with a Boat, a watercolor by Werner Gilles (1894-1961). The space between the figures is vibrant with feeling.

143

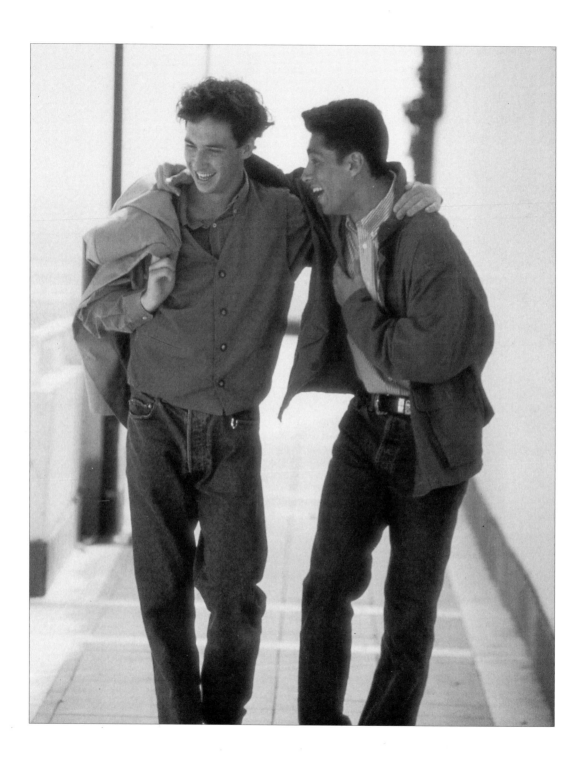

his willing slave. Some relationships of this type have been known to last a lifetime. But in spiritual terms both men have enslaved themselves: one to dominance, which corrupts the soul; and the other to slavery, which shrinks the soul. Sexual congress between such people is a mere ritual which satiates the flesh but cannot satisfy the mind. To be one or the other of such a pair indicates a psychological obsession which constantly disappoints because it never fulfills. Both roles stem from insecurity and low self-esteem.

The way out of such inequality is to bring pleasure, relaxation and laughter into the role playing. Break the mold. Allow the slave to become a clown and the master to become a kitten.

If in the first few weeks the new relationship seems equal, full of mutual interest and a fervent desire to be with one another, the next step is to spend a few days together. A weekend perhaps or a short holiday to relax and enjoy yourselves; but be watchful, too. Notice whether the common chores are shared. Do not let him take them all on his shoulders, nor should you bear the responsibility for making decisions on what to do, or where to go. Share all the decisions; never allow one partner to forfeit them.

If after a few months you realize that the time you are apart is flat and stale, without any spark of joy, it is time for momentous decisions. To join together may mean living together. Combining two male households and lives can be difficult, though; there are alternatives. You can spend half the time living together and half the time apart; or you can rent out one home, with the proviso that one of you can always return to it.

Do not overload the first few months with expectations, for often these will be doomed to disappointment. The first quarrel will seem like the end of the world. Do not overburden the relationship with ideas of what it should be like, or what should happen, or how your partner should behave. Go into the relationship with an open mind, heart, and soul. Be ready to experience everything afresh. Expect nothing and you will be rewarded a thousandfold.

Opposite: Early days. Full of mutual interest and a desire to be together.

HOW TO RECOGNIZE ONE IN LOVE

Sometimes one or other of a potential partnership is slow to realize that he is in love. He may feel a spark of interest for the other but have such low self-esteem that he does not recognize the first flowering of love within himself, nor can he see a reflected interest in the other.

Two of the signs of love are moodiness and restlessness. Those in love change quickly from being happy and ecstatic to being downcast and tearful. They are not able to stay quiet or sit still for many seconds, or else they lose their temper over something very trivial. They show discontent with their life, expressing their distaste about how they look, the way their hair grows, their weight, their size. Men in love get irritable about their clothes, job and hobbies, saying how much they hate something which everyone knows they have loved for years. They are impatient with every task, leaving things half done. They shut themselves up in their rooms for long periods. They play music very loudly. If told how strangely they are behaving, they deny it. They say with all honesty that they are behaving quite normally, as they always have done, and that nothing is the matter.

But if the name of their secret love is mentioned in conversation, a change is immediately apparent in them. They fall silent, eager to catch every word. And if the conversation continues on a different matter, they attempt to bring it back to their secret lover.

But what if this secret love object walks into the room? The one in love becomes nervous, falters on words, blushes, or goes so quiet he seems rooted to the spot, or else his voice changes into a higher register, and he begins to talk nonsense very quickly, spilling drinks, dropping objects and falling over feet. You would think the love object could not possibly miss such signs, but he may also be much in love and too busy trying to hide the fact.

In such cases, friends should try to save the couple, taking each aside to point out that the other is really interested in him. Once each of them is reassured and begins to believe that the potential lover feels something too, all is well. A thousand comedies, plays and novels have taken this theme as their inspiration and yet still lovers continue to behave as if they are totally ignorant of the elementary signs of love.

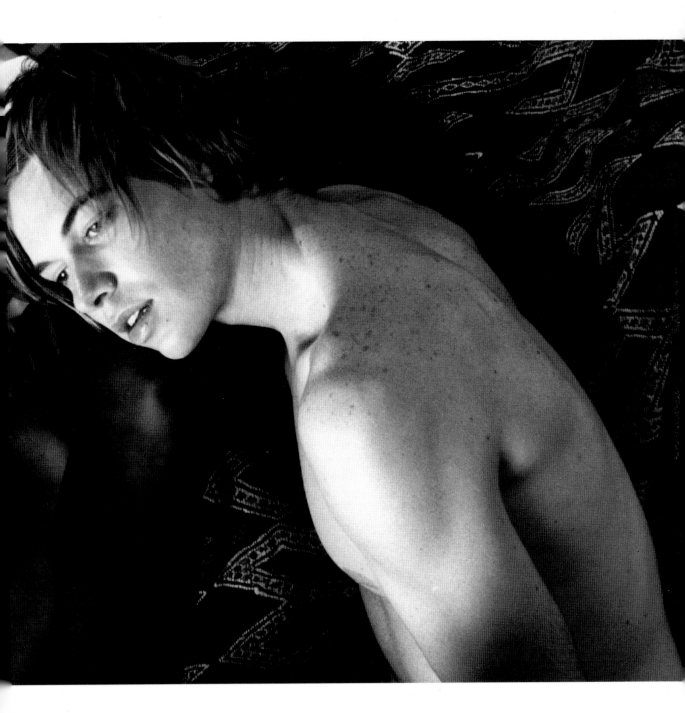

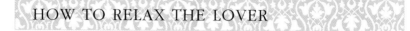

HOW TO RELAX THE LOVER

The best way to relax your lover is not to overload him with your own expectations. The relevance of this to the intimate side of a loving relationship cannot be over-emphasized. If a lover senses an anticipated requirement as to how he should behave, perhaps a tacit requirement that is never voiced but is simply there, it will engender fear and fright in him.

Be sensitive to his wishes. If you are both of one mind and you are sensitive to each other, a natural flow of sexual loving will develop. However, if your lover is tense and refuses to give any reason for it or honestly does not know the cause, you can pursue several paths.

Stop remarking on his state, and ignore the tension entirely. If he does not want to talk about it, leave it alone. Get on with your own work and your own interests. In the midst of these, provide small amusements for him. Ask his opinion on some mixture of fruit for a cordial. See if he likes a new recipe, or a canapé. But do not irritate him, and keep very cool. If he continues in the same bad state, leave him by himself for some hours, and while you are out buy him a small present. Keep to this routine for days if necessary.

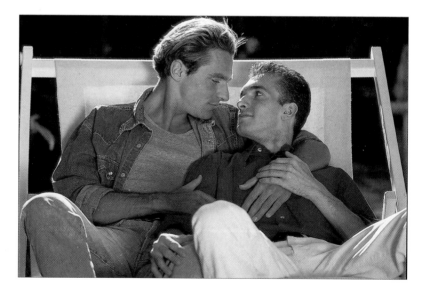

Mutual trust in a loving relationship.

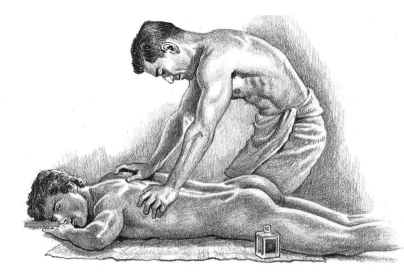

Massage. The perfect way
to relax your partner.

If he remains tense, change your tactics. Tell him that you are fed up with his bad moods and solitariness, and that he has to snap out of it or else threaten the whole relationship. Tell him what his mood is doing to your own happiness. Demand that he be truthful, however hurtful he thinks the truth might be.

This will nearly always produce a result. The cause of the tension may have been his inability to tell you the truth. Be ready to accept that it may be the end of the relationship.

Thankfully, a happier scenario is just as likely. If your lover longs to unwind, various practical steps can be taken. First, a small glass of champagne, second a warm bath, third a massage.

If he does not drink alcohol of any kind, a cool glass of iced camomile or peppermint tea with a dash of lime juice or angostura bitters is excellent for reviving the spirits. While he drinks it, sit next to him, take off his shoes and socks, place his feet on your lap and massage them. Work from the ankle downwards, treat each toe separately, gently bending and flexing, massage the sole and then up again towards the ankle. You can do this massage without oils. Then get up and prepare a bath perfumed with strong and heady aromas. While the water is running, stand behind his head and massage his neck and shoulders.

Help him undress and get into the bath. Dim the lighting. Play restful music softly in the background. Leave him to relax for ten to fifteen minutes, warm a large bath towel and choose some massage oils. Then help him out of the bath, wrap him around with the towel and dry him in front of a fire or somewhere warm. Prepare your essential oils (see page 174), place the towel on the floor and lay him on his stomach.

Start the massage with his neck and shoulders, moving on to his back and backbone, and then his upper arms down to his elbows. Massage down to the base of the backbone and to each side of the loins and the pelvic bones. Then move to his thighs, the backs of his knees and calves, then the ankle bones. Turn him over on to his back. Go back to the neck muscles and the shoulders, spend time on the rib cage and the chest, then move to his thighs, legs and feet. When you have finished, wrap him in a dry towel and let him sleep, or rest undisturbed, for at least half an hour.

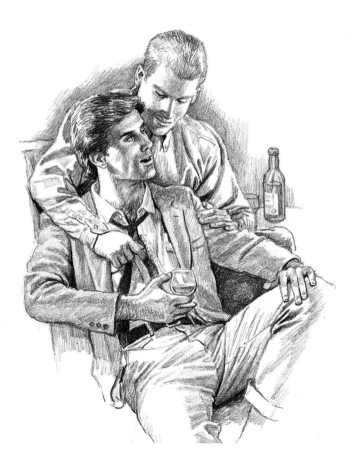

Seduction should be gentle and subtle; never go too far too quickly ...

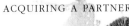

ON SEDUCTION

If the man you love is inexperienced and shy, if indeed he is a virgin who feels helpless and confused as to what to do, then you must proceed with caution and discretion.

At the first meeting merely touch and stroke his hands, telling him how beautiful, how talented, how charming and how very attractive he is. Then softly touch his face, his cheeks, even brush his lips and ear lobes. At this stage he will be more interested in the words of love than the action.

At the second meeting you may continue with the same, but this time brush your lips against his, and cover his cheek and neck with soft, feathery kisses. Make sure that your breath smells clean and sweet. Play with his hair and kiss the back of his neck.

On the third meeting you may continue to kiss and playfully use your tongue inside his mouth; then you may unbutton his shirt and stroke his chest, concentrating eventually upon his nipples, stroking them very gently so that they rise up, and planting kisses upon them. If you see that he is aroused, ask him if he is quite certain that he wants to continue. His own behavior will make this plain more than words can, as he begins to kiss you with an abandon he has never shown before.

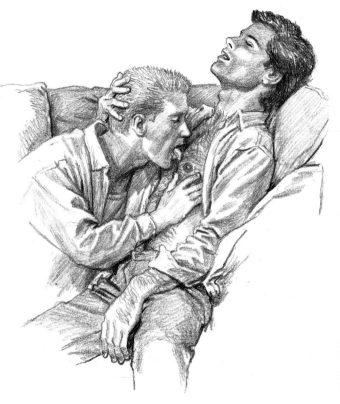

...take time undressing, and with every loving technique ...

But if this is not so, the love-making should end, however difficult it is for you. If he shows doubts and is hesitant, do not coerce. Let him return to his home and ponder on what has already happened. He will probably think of you with earnest sentiment which will turn to the most urgent desire in his loneliness. He will come to the fourth meeting desirous of all you want.

Now start where you left off. Kiss with tongues and arouse him by stroking and sucking his nipples. Take time with this art. Be patient in your industry. Lightly stroke and tickle the nipples with the tip of your

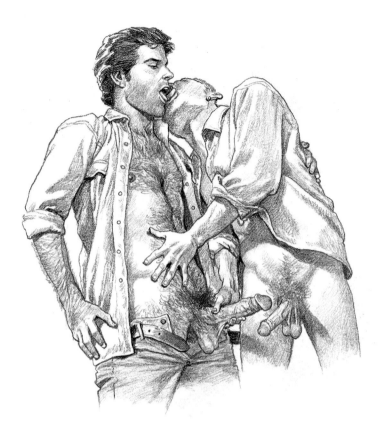

kiss with abandon, and lose
all sense of time and place.

tongue. The sensation a man will experience from this love-play is
immense. All sorts of ecstatic shudders will ripple through his body
from his groin to his lips. The size of his nipples will provide no indi-
cation of the ecstasy gained from their arousal. Any man can enter
paradise if his nipples are lovingly tended.

Then start to undress each other and embrace so that you may feel
each other's hot, naked skin pressing hard together. When you are
both naked, stretch out against each other and embrace. Give long
kisses with your tongue, nibbling and licking his ear lobes, then insert
your tongue into his inner ear, then withdraw and exhale hot breath
close to the ear. Let him feel your hard cock tight between his legs.
You must press hard so that your cock will touch and stroke that highly erotic part between the base of the scrotum and his anus. Then
change position and let him feel his cock in that same place on your

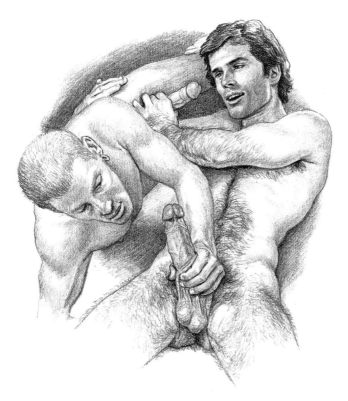

Sixty-nine, one of the most
pleasurable sexual experiences.

body. Your excitement may now be so charged that all you want is for
both of you to reach orgasm by rubbing on each other's bodies, or by
one of you coming between the other's tightly closed thighs. Coming
by rubbing on the belly is called "frottage." Coming between the
thighs is called "intercrural" and "interfemoral" sex.

In a new relationship, and especially with an inexperienced young
man, it is wise to leave penetration until last. Fellatio is a sexual activity generally enjoyed by both partners in the early days, and should
be part of the exploration of each other's bodies, not the means by
which orgasm is achieved unless this is plainly desired. Let each of
you take the other's cock into your mouth and feel its weight and
strength, taste the length of the shaft, then tentatively lick around the
rim of the knob with almost feathery touches of the tongue. Enclose
most of his cock with your hand, massaging it as it enters your mouth.

153

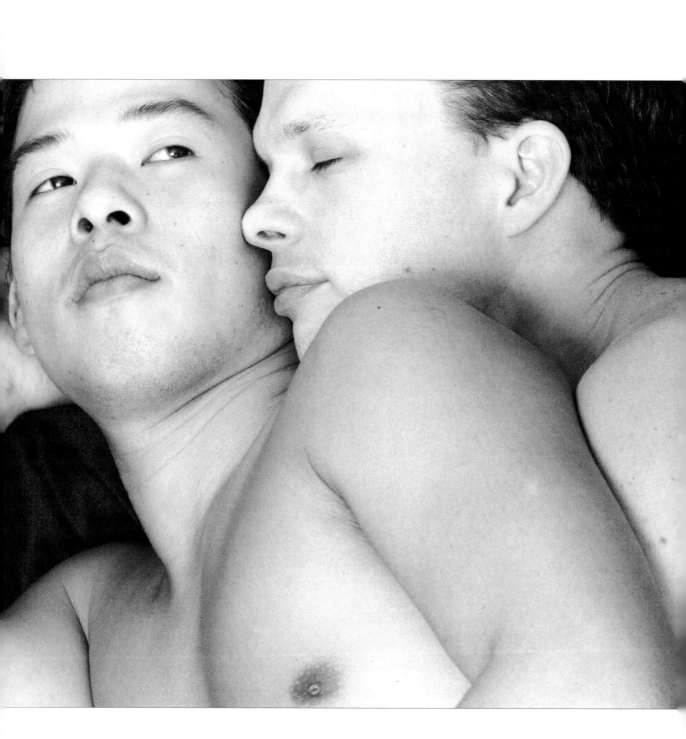

Use your saliva as a lubricant, sweeping the knob with your tongue.

After this highly arousing foreplay, you will want to fuck each other. If your lover is a virgin, he might very well feel quite nervous at the prospect, though longing for it and wanting to please you. Certain essential preliminaries are necessary before proceeding (see earlier sections on the subject, especially on penetration). You will need to guide him into an exploration of his anal orifice. Ensure that he is scrupulous in his hygiene. Tell him how to use enemas and allow him to explore your anus. Show him that if he oils his finger and very lightly massages the orifice and enters only a fraction, he will cause many shuddering sexual responses in your body. He should learn the importance of the sensitivity of this whole area, and in seeing your delight should also want to experience his own.

When the time is right, arrange him, with many kisses and embraces, on his back with his legs raised and open wide, so that he can see what you are doing. Tell him that for the moment you are going to devote all your attention to this often dismissed sexual organ so that he can decide which is the most pleasurable part of his body. Start by washing him with great care, using a perfumed soap and working up a great lather so that your hand and fingers are smooth and creamy. Wash inside him as well, then rinse with hot sponges and washcloths. Then change your position so that your own cock is over his head and he can suck it if he wishes (this is the position known as sixty-nine). Start licking between the scrotal sac and the anus, lick the crevice between the buns, and lastly lick the anus itself, letting your tongue first enter and then dart in and out. Using a perfumed oil, stroke and massage the same areas where your tongue has been, working two or three fingers into his anus and then allowing them to stay there for a moment or two. Then ask him to help you smooth a condom over your hard prick. Lubricate the condom well with a water-soluble jelly before resting the end of your cock against his anus and pressing gently.

After all that attention it is unlikely that he will suffer any pain on entry. If he does, stop thrusting but stay inside him so that he gets used to it. Practice will refine the art and make you both proficient at fucking each other with grace and elegance.

Opposite: Sleep and thoughtfulness, the post-coital feeling of unity and trust.

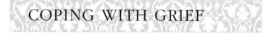

COPING WITH GRIEF

Bereavement can happen at any age; particularly now in the era of AIDS, devastating grief strikes the very young and those in their prime as well as the old. We all have to learn to cope. How can we go on living when we feel that part of us has gone into oblivion? How can we be in places that constantly remind us of our loss, of a partner who took delight in a particular scene or view? How can we hear a piece of music or listen to a poem which was a favorite of his? Worst of all, though, is the empty bed which once offered comfort and warmth. The unbearable reality of his loss chokes you with grief nightly.

You must battle alone with all the chores that together the pair of you had coped with effortlessly. You will need reserves of strength and many friends. Do not be too proud to accept company and invitations to visit, to stay over for weekends and to go out to dinner parties, concerts or the theater. You may not want to go out, but force yourself to. To stay in and grieve endlessly is pure self-indulgence. If you insist on doing it, you may be left without friends.

You will need to call on hidden reserves of strength to survive the days and nights. The first three months are the worst. Get through them—even by the skin of your teeth—and you'll be all right in the end. Life is for living; a great deal more fun remains for all of us, even after a devastating loss. We must learn how to be enriched by our suffering. Grief has the potential to deepen our knowledge of the human condition, reveal more to us about our own psychology and ultimately increase our capacity for enjoyment.

Such loss does not automatically signal the end of your love life, either. However remote the idea might seem in the early days of your grief, there will come a time when the sound of a voice or the glimpse of a face will rekindle a spark within you and a new relationship will beckon.

A lover who leaves causes another type of grief. If we are not careful this grief can destroy us, because the departed lover can destroy our self-worth and shatter our self-esteem, leaving us to fall into a pit of self-pity and loathing. We hate him and we hate ourselves for still loving him, for still wanting him.

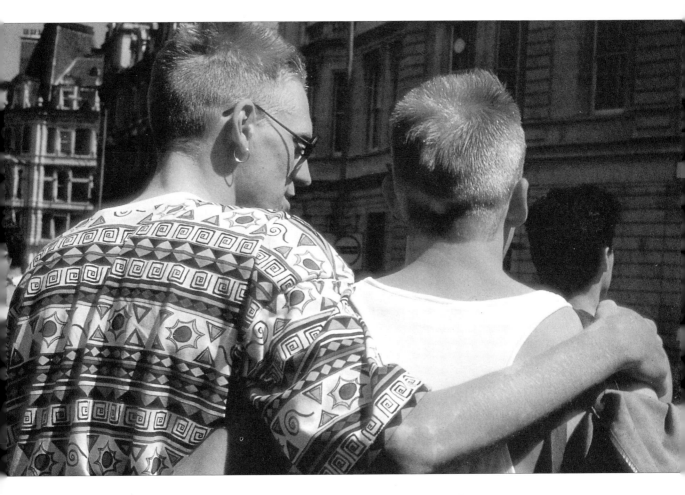

Though friends can sometimes help in this situation, more often than not they are a hindrance. Often they will happily participate in a group bitching session against your ex, but this will just allow you to sink more deeply into self-indulgence. Friends are more helpful with analyzing the reasons for his departure and getting a final perspective on what was wrong with the relationship. You will probably come to realize that the fault was not necessarily yours at all.

The best antidote to loss of self-esteem is a new, young, beautiful lover. A golden fuck will go a long way to wiping out the bad memories. And why stop at one?

HOW TO MANAGE ALONE

No man should live alone for long, yet there are periods when we have to for reasons beyond our control. There are times when no partner will even begin to fit into our lives. In these periods we tend to roam, wander and search, trying different people as if they were clothing, wondering whether this type or that one will fit. We may have many lovers.

The primary rules to follow in these periods concern your physical health and its preservation. Eat sparingly and select your food with care; lots of fresh raw vegetables and fruits, pasta and carbohydrates; no junk foods, meat or dairy products, which are full of saturated fats that will clog up your arteries. (Contrary to popular belief, milk is not a healthy food. All the calcium you need can be obtained from vegetables, preferably eaten raw, as cooking them can destroy their vitamin content.) Exercise regularly. Take care over personal hygiene and always practise safe sex. When picking up a partner, trust your instinct and act on it.

If you have been forced into having sex alone or started to prefer it, you will already have discovered which sexual aids are to your taste. There is a huge range of soft and hard porn magazines, videos, and a wide range of dildoes and leather aids to choose from. When you masturbate, be sure not to restrict your breathing or block the flow of blood to the brain. Such activities are dangerous and can lead to death.

CHANGING PARTNERS

Love does not remain the same: like everything else it grows and changes. Some aspects of love can die. If one partner is very young at the onset of the affair, it is not unusual for him to outgrow the relationship. Both partners may realize that their feelings for each other have faded. When a love affair began with such passion and high hopes, it can be difficult to face the fact that it has changed irrevocably over the years. Of course, in many cases a partnership can still be saved because there is something durable and good at its very center.

Opposite: Companionship can last a lifetime.

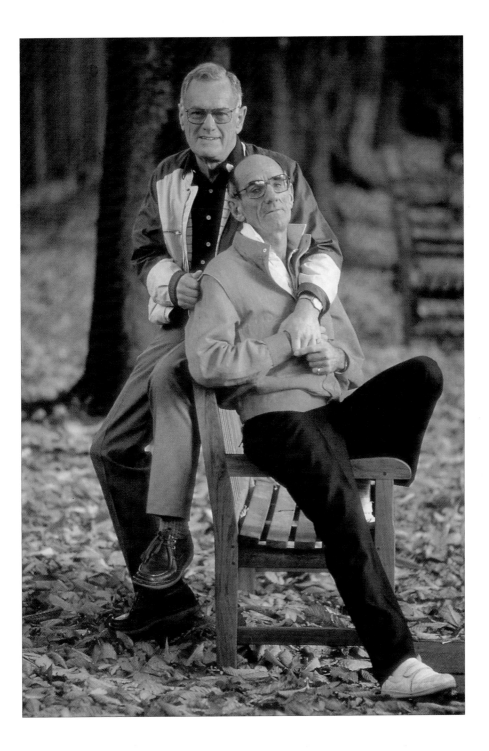

However, if sexual passion has died, consider carefully what the future holds. You both might want to stay together but have an open relationship. If you agree to do so, it is extremely important to practise safe sex at all times.

In opening the relationship to other partners, you may meet someone with whom you fall in love and want to change partners altogether. This situation can cause much pain. The people involved may become bitter. The one in love may believe he can never leave his partner because the break would be too hurtful. I have known men allow this belief to keep them in a sterile relationship for years. The truth is that people are survivors and fear of hurting someone deeply should not halt your own development or blight your chance for future happiness.

Often it is best to make a clean break; leave quickly and explain that practical arrangements, such as splitting property (a highly sensitive subject), can be dealt with later. This at least has the merit of decisiveness. The partner you have left has to cope with the fact that you really have gone and it avoids endless discussions over the physical arrangements of leaving.

If you have been together for many years and split everything fairly, fewer problems arise. All the objects and furniture brought into the relationship should be kept by each owner, and everything bought while living together should be divided equally between you.

In reality, however, people's lives are rarely that equal. One partner may be richer than the other, or have a stable income while the other's income fluctuates. Perhaps one partner has paid more and even owns the apartment. In this matter the best solution is to follow the heterosexual model, which recognizes that women who are not wage earners bring their skill, time and creative gifts into the home over the years entitling them to some financial gain when it is sold. This principle is rarely acknowledged in gay relationships. It may be possible to find a gay lawyer to pursue a settlement along these lines.

The best solution lies with the partners themselves. If each can be both modest and generous in his demands upon the other at such a time, then the relationship has some chance of enduring, albeit on a different basis from that originally conceived for it. An ex-partner's friendship is very much worth keeping.

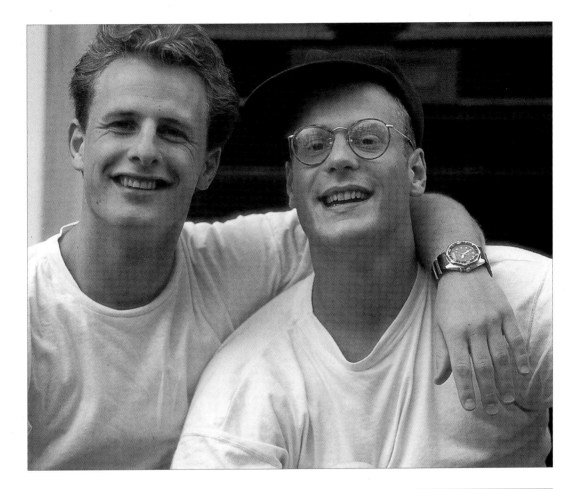

Self-esteem, consideration and trust
form the basis of lasting love.

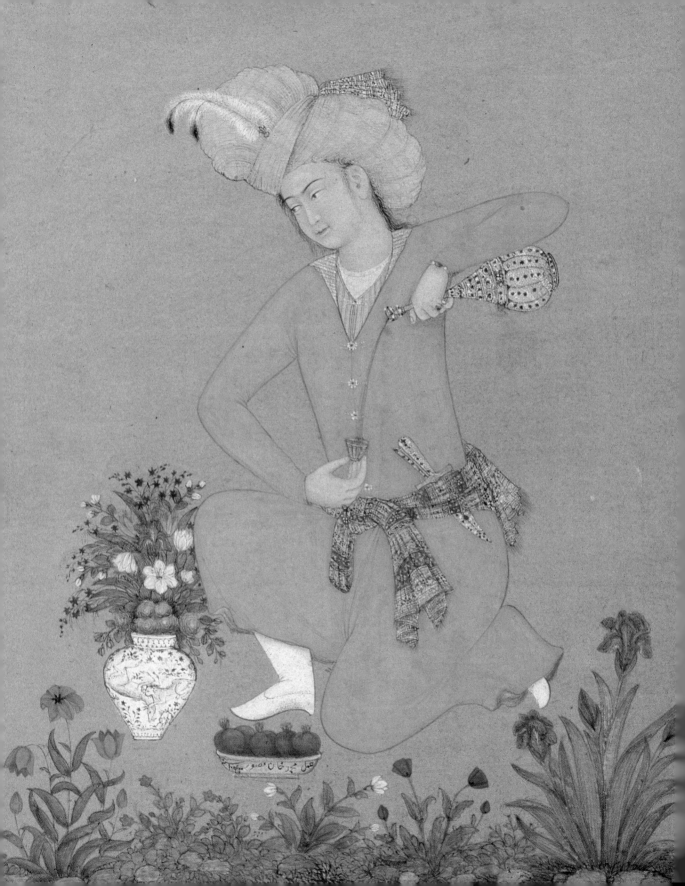

CHAPTER SIX
STIMULANTS AND RELAXANTS

When a man wishes to enlarge his lingam, he should rub it with the bristles of certain insects that live in trees, and then, after rubbing it for ten nights with oils, he should again rub it with the bristles as above. By continuing to do this a swelling will be gradually produced in the lingam, and he should then lie on a cot and cause his lingam to hang through a hole in the cot. After this he should take away all the pain from the swelling by using cool concoctions. The swelling, which is called "Suka" and is often brought about among the people of the Dravida country, lasts for life. If the lingam is rubbed with the following things: the plant physalis flexuosa, the shavara-kandaka plant, the jalasuka plant, the fruit of the egg plant, the butter of a she-buffalo, the hasti-charma plant, and the juice of the vajra-rasa plant, a swelling lasting for one month will be produced. By rubbing it with oil boiled in the concoctions of the above things, the same effect will be produced, but lasting for six months. The enlargement of the lingam is also effected by rubbing it or moistening it with oil boiled on a moderate fire along with the seeds of the pomegranate and the cucumber, the juices of the valuka plant, the hasti-charma plant and the egg plant....The people in the southern counties have also a congress in the anus that is called the "lower congress."

True love and its sensual celebration can be enhanced with either a stimulant or a relaxant. *The Kama Sutra* explores both. The ancient world believed in aphrodisiacs with a great fervor, which may have made many of them work. Some people swear by aphrodisiacs today, but the romantic context in which they are used, rather than the substances themselves, may give them their arousing effect. Imagine a candle-lit meal with soft, background music, subtly seasoned dishes and the air full of heady, spicy aromas. Such a combination would be enough to lull anybody into a sensual state.

Opposite: Persian prince pouring wine. An Indian miniature from 1633-42.

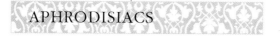

APHRODISIACS

Here is a list of some of the most familiar aphrodisiacs that are non-toxic and can be used safely, as foods, herbs and perfumes:

Almonds: ground and mixed with cream, stock and egg yolk to make a soup.

Ambergris: a heavenly perfumed substance, secreted from the intestines of the sperm whale found in tropical seas. Madame du Barry supposedly used ambergris as a perfume to retain the affection of Louis XV.

Anise: can be eaten whole or its seeds crushed and used to flavor other dishes.

Aromatic bath: an indispensable preliminary to seduction among the Romans, it was followed by a massage with all manner of perfumed unguents. (See Aromatherapy, page 26.)

Artichoke: in France the globe variety was always regarded as a powerful aphrodisiac. Catherine de Medici ate quantities of them. The cry of Parisian street vendors selling them was that they were hot for the genitals.

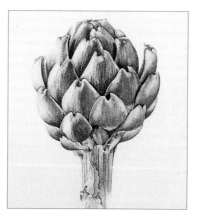

Artichoke study, by
Alison Cooper.

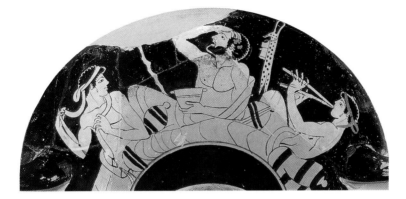

Drinking scene painted on a
Greek bowl, fifth century B.C.

Asparagus: a great favorite of the ancient Romans, and also among the Arabs who believed that a daily dish of asparagus produced all the erotic effect anyone could want.

Basil: a favored aromatic plant in India and elsewhere. According to a nineteenth-century physician, basil "helps the deficiency of Venus."

Capsicum annuum: this sweet pepper, which is the main ingredient of paprika, can be used as a condiment, sprinkled on food or put into sauces and stews.

Caraway: another favorite spice of the ancients, and one that is frequently mentioned in Oriental love manuals.

Cardamom: these tiny black and highly aromatic seeds can be pounded together with ginger and cinnamon and sprinkled over foods.

Celery: a favorite way to begin a meal in eighteenth-century France was to have celery made into a soup.

Chocolate: in the seventeenth century monks were forbidden to drink chocolate because of its reputed effect.

165

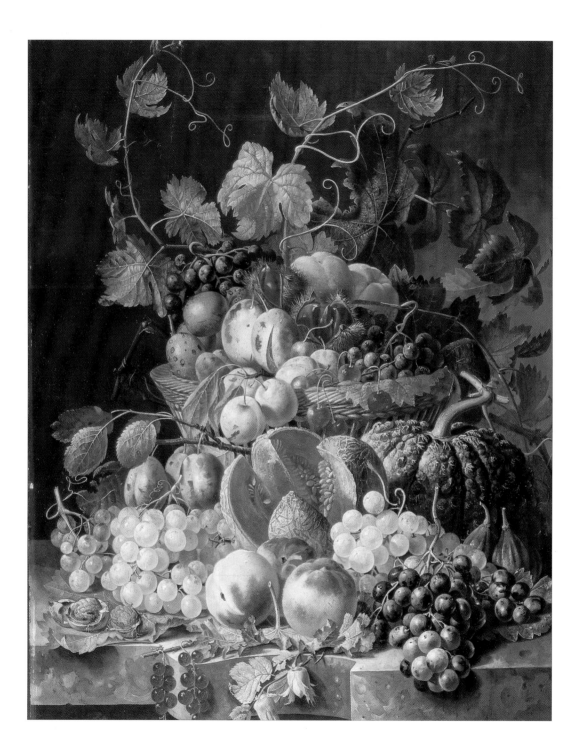

Cinnamon: mentioned for its erotic properties in *The Song of Songs* (4.14).

Coriander: this has to be gathered in the last quarter of the Moon.

Cumin: the seeds of this highly aromatic plant are ground and used sprinkled over food or added to the cooking.

Egg yolk: long considered a stimulant in nearly all countries. *The Perfumed Garden* says that he who eats three egg yolks every day will be sexually invigorated.

Fennel: a Hindu recipe for sexual vigor includes the juice of the fennel plant with milk mixed with honey, ghee, liquorice and sugar.

Fig: always regarded as possessing highly stimulating properties. Figs played a prominent part in the Dionysia, festivals of the Greek god of wine and ecstasy, Dionysus.

Galingale: a spicy aromatic root treasured by the Indians. In an Arab recipe it is crushed with cardamoms, nutmeg, gillyflowers, cloves and Persian pepper, before adding water. The resultant brew is drunk night and morning.

Garlic: revered in ancient Japan, China, India, Greece and Egypt. Use two heads of garlic to make a soup, thicken with almonds, flavor with saffron.

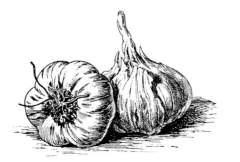

Opposite: Basket of Fruit, by Johannes Hendrick Fredriks (1774-1822).

Left: Heads of garlic.

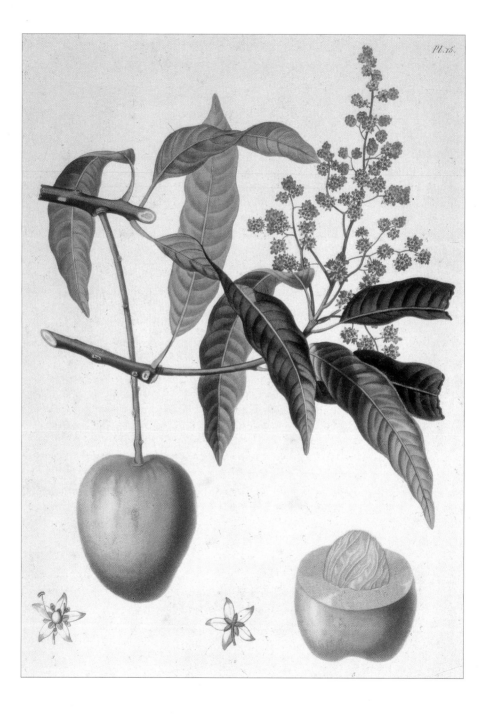

Pl.15.

Ginger: appears as a vital ingredient in Turkish, Indian, Arabian and Chinese love recipes.

Ginseng: long thought to have erotic properties.

Honey: appears as an ingredient in many recipes for love potions.

Juniper: the berries produce an oil which is supposed to maintain youthful ardor. Juniper is used as a flavoring; gin, for example, is flavored with it.

Mango: a Hindu favorite; the fruit and juice were used, as was the stone, from which an oil used as an ointment was extracted.

Mastic: pounded with honey and oil, this wonderfully aromatic substance from the mastic tree was thought to increase the amount of sperm.

Myrtle: can be taken internally and used externally. The leaves were crushed and applied to the genitals. A recipe for a cordial gives two handfuls of the flowers and leaves of the myrtle which are then distilled with two quarts of spring water and a quart of white wine for twenty-four hours.

Nutmeg: highly prized in the Orient, especially by Chinese women, and used to spice all kinds of foods.

Onion seed: A popular remedy mentioned in *The Perfumed Garden* has it pounded and mixed with honey.

Oyster: the one aphrodisiac food probably everyone has heard of. The ancient world was divided on the subject of its benefits. Ovid did not prize oysters, but Juvenal did.

Peach: together with the fig, the fruit most favored as a stimulant.

Opposite: Mango tree, from *Flore des Antilles,* 1808-27, by F. R. de Tussac.

169

Pepper: considered highly effective if ground with nettle seed.

Pistachio: this nut was frequently mentioned in Arab love manuals.

Rocket (*Eruca sativa*): one of the best known and most reliable of all aphrodisiacs, this salad green was eaten extensively in the ancient world. Thought to be sacred to the god Priapus, its seed was sprinkled around all statues dedicated to him. Columella, the Roman poet, wrote: "The eruca, Priapus, near thee we sow/To rouse to duty husbands who are slow." Rocket salad was recommended by both Ovid and Martial. The leaves were dressed with olive oil, vinegar, pepper and chopped garlic.

Saffron: according to a Greek legend, a girl who consumes saffron for a whole week will not be able to resist her lover.

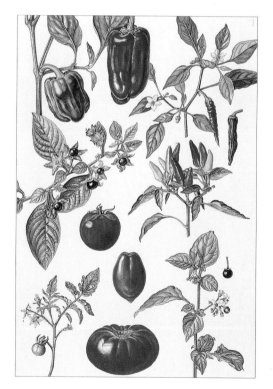

Right: Pepper and related fruits, by Elizabeth Rice.

Opposite: The Young Bacchus, by Caravaggio, *c.*1591-3.

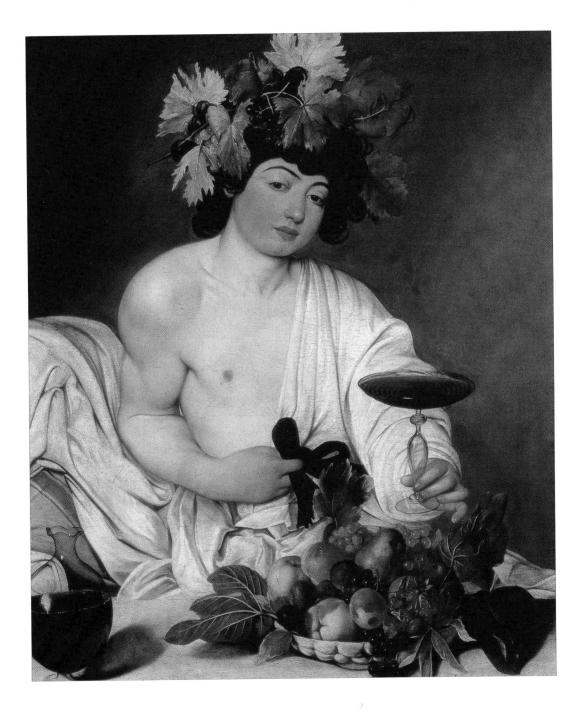

Sage: the juice from the pounded leaves should be mixed with honey.

Tarragon: use the leaves to flavor salads.

Thyme: use in cooking.

Vanilla: Vanilla pods give a wonderful, heady aroma and flavor to dishes. Madame de Pompadour loved chocolates flavored with vanilla and ambergris. Leave a vanilla pod in a jar of sugar to flavor the contents.

Up to now there has been no scientific proof that the vast majority of the traditional aphrodisiacs are effective.

The two highly dangerous ones, which should in no circumstances be used, are Cantharides and Yohimbene.

Cantharides (*Lytta vesicatoria* or "Spanish Fly") is a species of beetle found in southern Europe. It has bright blue fluorescent wings and these, at least, will turn up in spice mixtures found in the markets of north Africa. The whole dried beetle is crushed into a powder and added to foods. The active substance, cantharides, irritates the genito-urinary tract to such a degree that any action like peeing or coming is a relief. Used in the East medicinally to burn off warts, it is highly toxic and contact with it can produce a blister. Taken internally it can cause kidney damage, severe gastro-enteritis, blood in the urine and death. Priapism is merely mentioned as a side symptom. Clearly, this is not a substance to play around with.

Yohimbene is derived from the bark of the Yohimbene tree, native to central Africa. The bark is boiled in water and the resultant liquor reduced before being drunk. A West Indian recipe mixes it with puréed aubergine, peppercorns, chillies, pimentos and vanilla. The bark contains strychnine, which is very dangerous.

Opposite: Rosemary and other herbs. Watercolor by Elizabeth Rice.

·Elizabeth H. Rice·

AYURVEDIC MEDICINE

The Kama Sutra is imbued with ideas from various classical Indian traditions. Ayurveda, the classical medical tradition of India, is one of these. The word *Ayurveda* comes from Sanskrit and means "Knowledge of long life." The Vedic literature of around 1500 B.C. produced by the Aryan people honored a vast number of gods, all of them highly sexual beings and each of whom governed some aspect of life or nature, such as the sun, sky, moon, dawn, wind, or fire. In Ayurvedic medicine the body is thought to be composed of five elements: earth, water, fire, wind and space. Each of these elements relates directly to an organ, a bodily fluid or a function, just as each of them relates to the wider world. The individual is therefore seen both as part of the universe and as a universe in himself.

A happy and healthy being is one who is truly balanced between the individual ego and the context in which he thrives. Ayurvedic medicine is a totally holistic concept which takes into account every aspect of a person (such as diet, sexuality, spirituality, physical well-being and emotions), as well as the natural and social environment in which he lives.

Ayurvedic remedies involve the use of various traditional therapies, including acupuncture, homeopathy, massage, osteopathy and herbalism. The essence and oils of various plants are used; favorite among these are ginger, pomegranate, licorice, myrrh, basil and garlic.

ESSENTIAL OILS

The history of essential oils goes back to at least 2000 B.C. The Chinese and the Egyptians were among the first to use them extensively. Valued for their antiseptic properties, essential oils were used as protection against plague. In the nineteenth century chemical copies of essential oils began to flood the market. These were cheaper to make but less powerful and not as therapeutic. Further investigation in the West revealed that essential oils penetrate the skin and are carried around in the circulatory system, reaching the blood and lymph. Thus, they can be used to cure many ailments, while

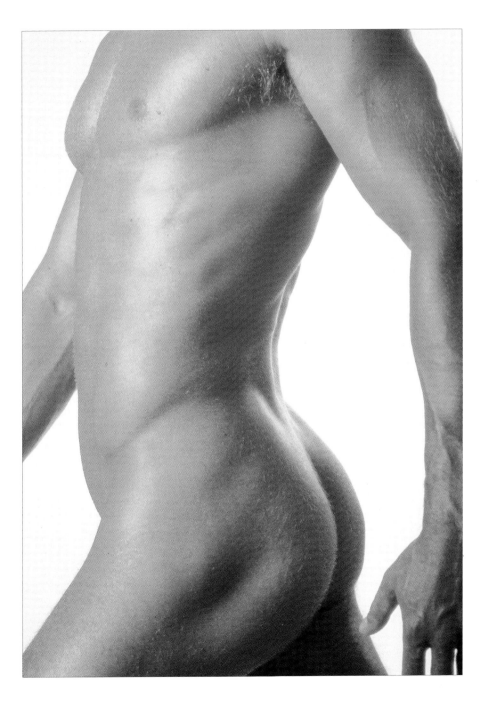

giving a sense of well-being that is incalculable. The time-scale in which essential oils begin to do their good work varies from person to person; with some individuals penetration into the circulation occurs within half an hour, with others it can take twelve hours.

All essential oils can be used in baths, in burners and as inhalants. However, when used for massage, as perfume or for skin care, they must be diluted in an odorless base or carrier oil. Corn, sunflower or grape seed oil would all do. You can create your own recipes by blending oils within the carrier oil.

The Principal Groups of Oils

There are three main groups of essential oils: those for the spirit, those that enhance the general health of the individual, and those that may be given as sedatives. Below you will find separate listings for each group. Please note that each essential oil has its own special properties and is suited to different applications. The information given below is intended as a guide only, so it is important that before using any of the oils listed you find out the correct amounts or dosages from a qualified source.

Quick-acting and uplifting oils:

Basil: used extensively in India. It will clear the head and give a great sense of well-being. Recommended for the digestion and nervous depression or hysteria.

Bergamot: this member of the citrus family is given for herpes (cold sores), skin blemishes such as acne or ulcers, and can cure bad breath and sore throats. It is used in eau de Cologne and lavender water and to flavor Earl Grey tea. It is a powerful antiseptic.

Clary sage: sometimes used in the making of German Muscatel wines and by the Italians in Vermouth. Also a component of eau de Cologne and lavender water. Recommended for high blood pressure and sore throats.

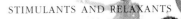

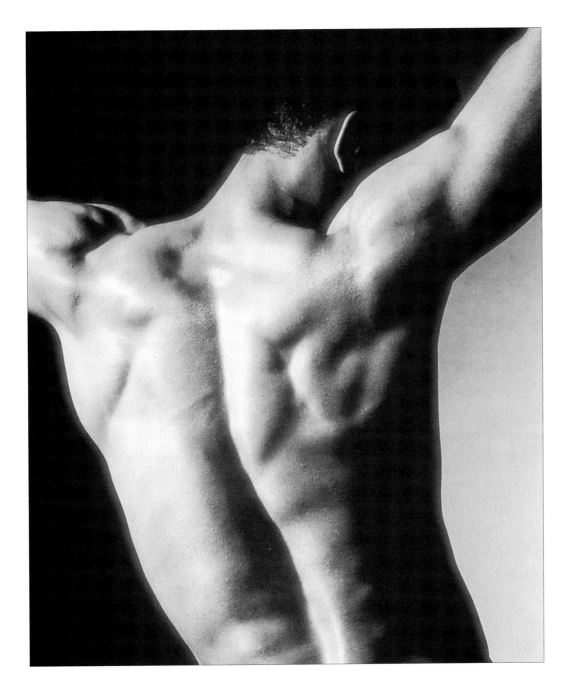

Eucalyptus: part of various commercial preparations used for rubbing on chests to improve breathing difficulties associated with colds. It is also good for diarrhea and for muscular aches and pains.

Lemon: the oil is obtained from the rind of the fruit. Lemon is given for circulatory and respiratory problems, high blood pressure and asthma. Excellent for greasy skin, herpes, insect bites and wrinkles.

Lemon grass: relieves indigestion and skin problems.

Sage: a diuretic that also soothes muscular pains and nervous conditions.

Oils for general metabolism:

Black Pepper: aids digestion, is a diuretic, and also helps with colds, toothache and muscular aches and pains. Can be rubbed on.

Camomile: an excellent digestive; good for liver disorders, loss of appetite, earache and toothache.

Cypress: energizes a sluggish circulation and helps clear coughs and colds.

Fennel: noted as a digestive; also used for colic, constipation, flatulence, nausea and vomiting.

Geranium: used for head, mouth and throat infections, and in the treatment of nervousness and depression; cleansing of the skin.

Hyssop: aid to circulatory, digestive and respiratory problems.

Opposite: Juniper, by Dr Woodville, 1793

Juniper: good for rheumatic pains, stress and insomnia.

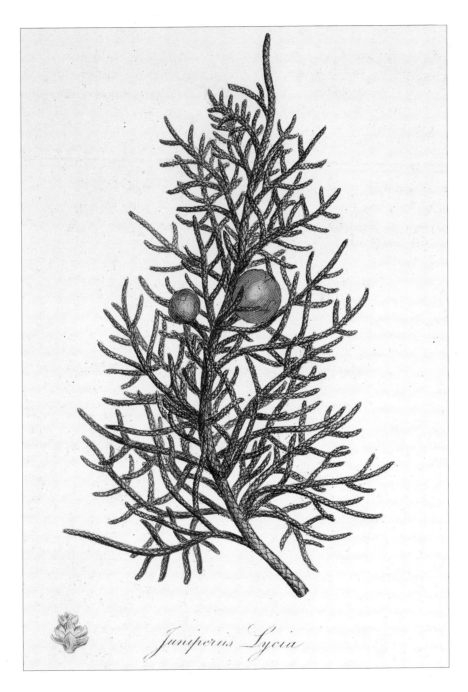

Juniperus Lycia

Lavender: treatment for high blood pressure, migraine and depression.

Marjoram: a general calmative; reduces irritability; also helps the effects of asthma.

Melissa: a digestive; given for nausea, shock and tension. Soothes bee and wasp stings.

Peppermint: stops diarrhea and stomach pains, bad breath and catarrh. Also used as an insect repellent.

Pine needle: given for gall stones and respiratory infections.

Rosemary: helps stomach pains, mental fatigue, migraine and general nervous debility.

Thyme: moves sluggish bowels; helps insomnia and catarrh.

Relaxing oils:

Camphor, cedarwood, frankincense, jasmine, marigold, myrrh, orange blossom, patchouli, rose, sandalwood.

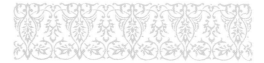

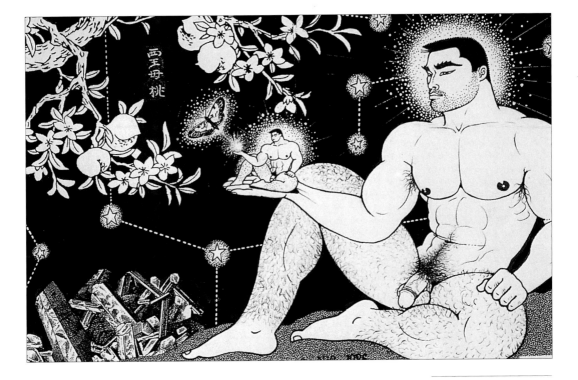

Dream of a Dream, ink drawing
by Sadao Hasegawa.

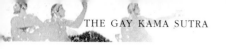

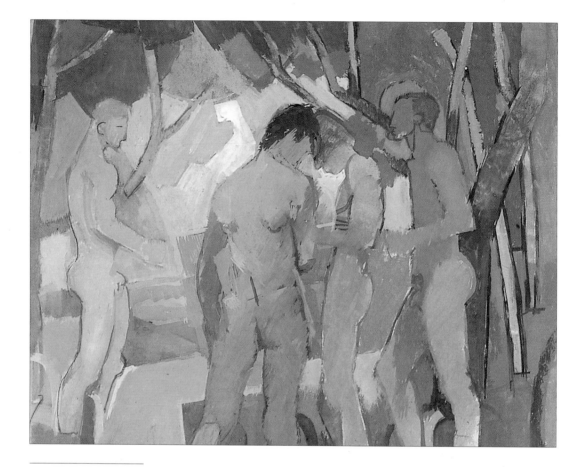

Bathers in a Wood, by
Cornelius McCarthy. A tribute
to both Cézanne and Keith
Vaughan, the painting shows
how traditional and enduring
the theme is.

FURTHER READING

Boswell, John. *Christianity, Social Tolerance and Homosexuality: Gay People in Western Europe from the Beginning of the Christian Era to the Fourteenth Century.* (Chicago: University of Chicago Press, 1980)

Bullough, Vern L. *Sexual Variance in Society and History.* (Chicago: University of Chicago Press, 1976)

Burton, Peter and Smith, Richard. *Vale of Tears: A Problem Shared.* (Brighton: Millevre Books, 1992)

Cantarella, Eva. *Bisexuality in the Ancient World.* Trans. C.O.O'Cuilleanain. (New Haven: Yale University Press, 1992)

Coote, Stephen (ed.). *The Penguin Book of Homosexual Verse.* (London: Penguin, 1983)

Dickens, Joy. *Family Outing: A Guide for Parents of Gays, Lesbians and Bisexuals.* (London: Peter Owen, 1995)

Dubermann, Martin. *About Time: Exploring the Gay Past.* (New York: Gay Presses of New York, 1986)

Harry, Joseph and DeVall, William B. *The Social Organization of Gay Males.* (New York: Praeger, 1978)

Hart, Jack (ed.). *My First Time.* (Boston: Alyson Press, 1995)

James, Trevor and others. *On the Safe Edge.* (Toronto: Whole S M Publishing, 1994)

Katz, Jonathan N. *Gay American History: Lesbians and Gay Men in the USA.* (New York: Crowell, 1976)

Lucas, Ian. *Growing Up Positive: Stories from a generation of young people affected by Aids.* (London: Cassell, 1995)

Marshall, Andrew. *Together Forever.* (London: Pan, 1995)

Romesburg, Don (ed.). *Young, Gay and Proud.* (Boston: Alyson Books, 1995)

Sanderson, Terry. *How to be a Happy Homosexual.* (London: The Other Way Press, 1995)

—— *A-Z of Gay Sex.* (London: The Other Way Press, 1994)

—— *Assertively Gay.* (London: The Other Way Press, 1993)

—— *A Stranger in the Family.* (London: The Other Way Press, 1996)

—— *Making Gay Relationships Work.* (London: The Other Way Press, 1995)

Signorile, Michelangelo. *Outing Yourself: How to come out as lesbian or gay to your family, friends and colleagues.* (London: Abacus, 1996)

Silverstein, Dr Charles and Picano, Felice. *The New Joy of Gay Sex.* (New York: HarperCollins, 1992)

Spencer, Colin. *Homosexuality in History.* (New York: Harcourt Brace and Co., 1996)

Sutcliffe, Lynn. *There Must be Fifty Ways to Tell Your Mother.* (London: Cassell, 1996)

Tatchell, Peter. *Safer Sexy : The Guide to Gay Sex Safely.* (London: Freedom Editions/Cassell, 1994)

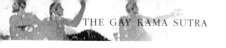

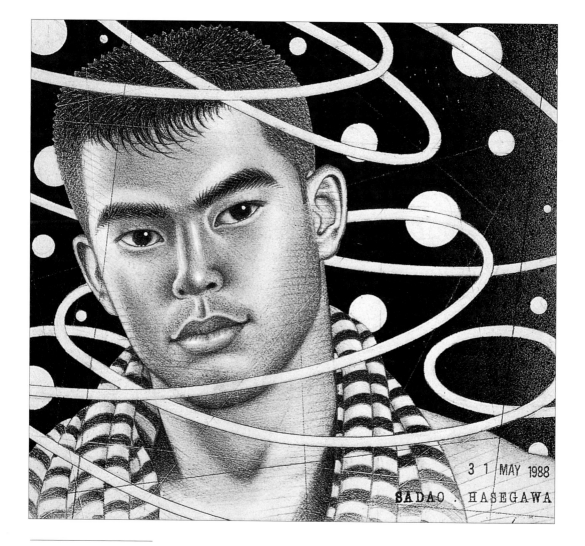

Untitled II, by Sadao Hasegawa.

INDEX

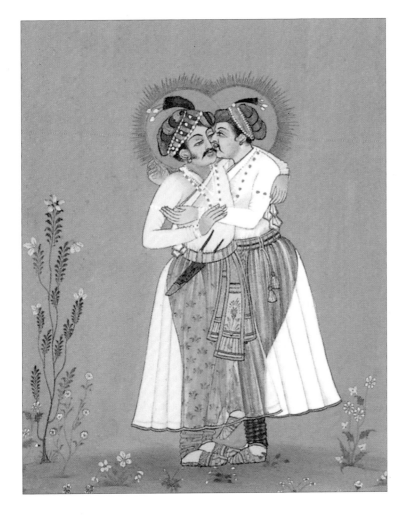

A contemporary miniature
in the Mughal tradition.

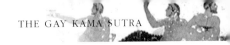

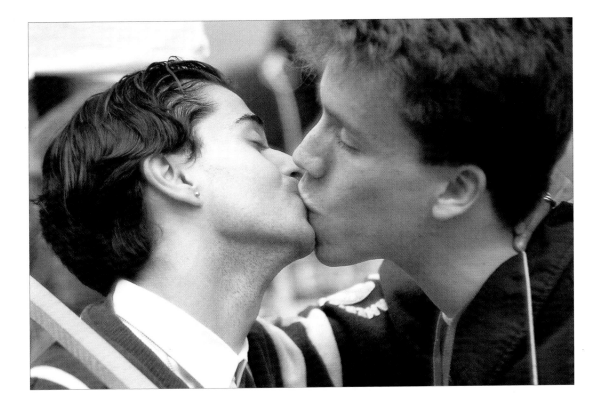

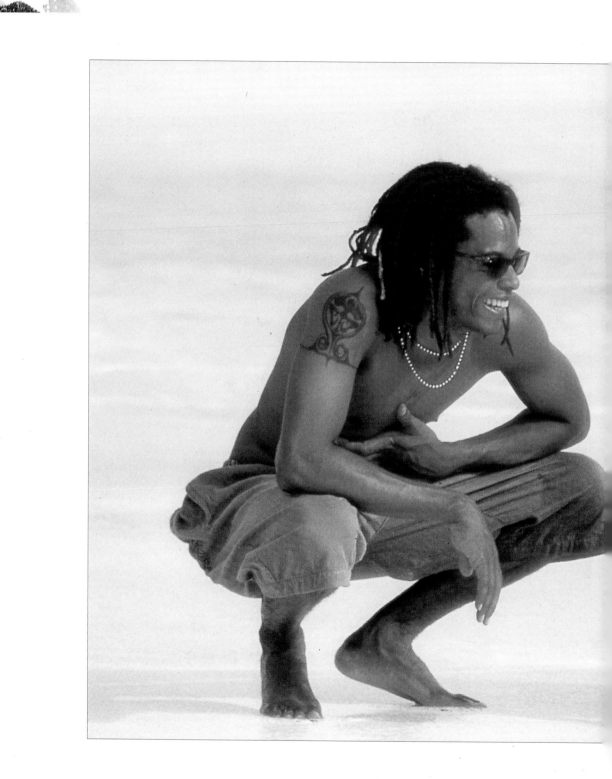

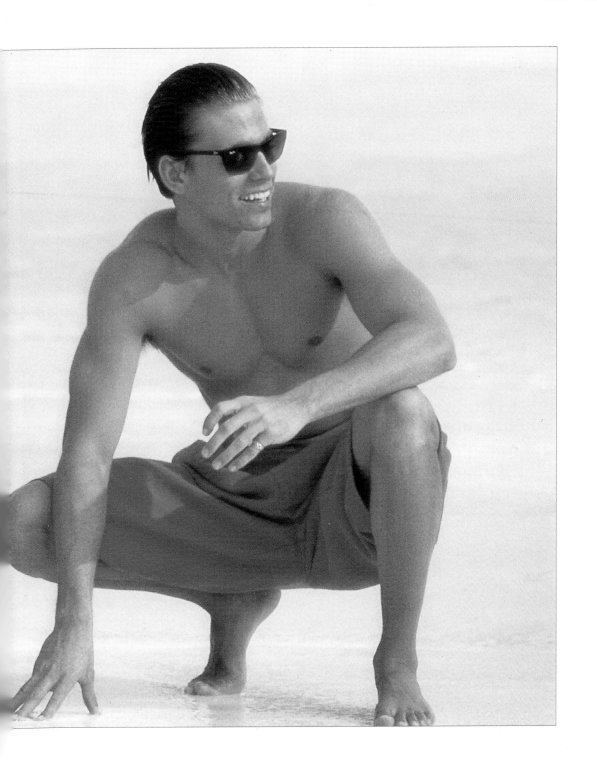

ACKNOWLEDGMENTS

Commissioned drawings by Roger Payne/Linden Artists (London): 41, 43, 44, 45, 46, 48, 49, 54, 56, 57, 59, 60, 61, 64, 68, 69, 87, 124, 128, 149, 150, 151, 152, 153

Picture research by Image Select International (London)
AKG: 162 (India Office Library, London)
Alison Cooper: 164 (Private Collection)
Ancient Art & Architecture Collection: All running heads, 79, 89
Ann Ronan/Image Select: 105, 167
The Bridgeman Art Library: 23, 179
British Library, London (The Bridgeman Art Library) : 168
British Museum, London (The Bridgeman Art Library): 27, 34
Chiartosini, P.P.: 9
E. T. Archive: 39, 123
Fitzwilliam Museum, Cambridge (The Bridgeman Art Library): 166
Format Photographers Ltd: 77 and 159 Val Wilmer; 81 and 157 Pam
    Isherwood; 99 Donna Binder; 103 and 116 Brenda Prince
Gabinetto dei Disegni e delle Stampe, Firenze (Scala): 95
GMP Publishers Ltd/Éditions Aubrey Walters, PO Box 247, Swaffham,
    Norfolk PE37 8PA:
    67, 72, 126, from the book *Private: The Erotic Art of Duncan Grant*
    by Douglas Blair Turnbaugh (1989)
    129, 130, 181, 184, from the book *Sadao Hasegawa* (1989)
Hoffman, David: 40, 42, 154, 189
The Image Bank (posed by models): Frontispiece, 31, 32, 37, 47, 98, 108,
    133, 144, 161, 177, 190, 191
Images Colour Library: 21
Katz, Tamara: Copyright page
Louvre Museum, Paris: 25, 28, 71
Louvre Museum, Paris (The Bridgeman Art Library): 18, 38, 94,
McCarthy, Cornelius: 85, 90, 182
Musée D'Orsay, Paris (The Bridgeman Art Library): 78, 110
Photofusion: 33; 96, 97, 101 and 113 David Montford; 137 Debbie Humphry
Pictor International: 148
Pinacoteca di Brera, Milan (Superstock): 51
Prado, Madrid (The Bridgeman Art Library): 82
Premgit: 12
Private Collections (The Bridgeman Art Library): 106, 170, 173
Réunion des Musées Nationaux, Paris: 19, 35 and 165 H. Lewandowski; 26
Rex Features: 115 (Stills), 117, 119
Simpson, Ron and Jay Patel: 15, 53, 58, 63, 187
Städtisches Museum, Mulheim (The Bridgeman Art Library): 142
Southern, Andrew, at So Dam Tuff: 147
Telegraph Colour Library: 29, 30, 76, 135, 141, 175
Thadani, Giti: 8, 14
Tretyakov Gallery, Moscow (Superstock): 74
Uffizi, Florence (The Bridgeman Art Library): 171
Victoria & Albert Museum, London (The Bridgeman Art Library): 6, 11, 92, 122
Whitford & Hughes (The Bridgeman Art Library): 86